Grow Up Without Getting Old!

Lifestyle Choices To Put Life Into Your Years & Years Into Your Life

D1519992

Salvatore Lacagnina, D.O.

Grow Up Without Getting Old!
Copyright ©2020 Salvatore Lacagnina, D.O.

Columns originally published in the *News-Press*. Reprinted with permission.

Cover Design: MAF Marketing & Design
Cover Graphic: ©Fisher Photostudio
Library of Congress Control Number: 2018675309
Printed in the United States of America

ISBN 979-8-5751-2528-0

Advanced Praise

"Dr. Sal's dedication to lifestyle medicine and his book are inspiring evidence that you, not medicines and machines, can control your health. Live long and love the journey!"

- **Dr. Michael Greger, MD FACLM, Founder of NutritionFacts.org, Author of *How Not To Die***

"This book is a healthy 'all-you-can-eat buffet' of science-backed information that will transform your health one bite at a time. Dr. Sal masterfully weaves together in each chapter the perfect blend of science, wisdom, humor and practical answers to important questions. It is ideal for the kitchen table or nightstand and deserves to be read more than once."

- ***Dr. Scott Stoll, MD FABPMR, Co-Founder The Plantrician Project***

"Using the six pillars of lifestyle medicine in everyday life will help people to enjoy life with vitality, energy, and robust health."

- ***Dr. Elizabeth Pegg Frates, MD, Lifestyle Medicine Specialist ; Health & Wellness Coach***

"Dr. Sal addresses the most common health concerns we all face, giving research-informed educational bites imbued with his sage advice, his heart, and inspiration. An article a day from Dr. Sal will help you keep disease and the hospital away! This book is a must-read for those interested in optimizing their health and aging."

   - **Dr. Cate Collings, President of American College of Lifestyle Medicine**

"Dr. Sal is a leading light in Lifestyle Medicine."

   - Dr. Darren Morton, PhD, Director of the Lifestyle Medicine and Health Research Centre, Avondale University College

Dedication

I dedicate this book to the beautiful, little red headed child that I met early in the 1980s when I was completing a college internship.

As part of the internship, I spent time at the Association for Children with Down Syndrome (ACDS) on Long Island, New York. This is where I met Andy who subsequently changed the direction of my life. Andy had Down syndrome, a disease I was very familiar with as several of my family members had the same.

My time at the Association was spent working with Andy during the school year and at the end of the semester his parents asked me to work with him during the summer because the school was closed during this time.

I was honored to do this and enjoyed every moment taking Andy to the park, having lunch with him and seeing him grow as a young child.

I started reading and learning more about Down syndrome which led me to read about other hereditary disorders and then other medical topics.

As a result of this curiosity and new learning, I made the decision to apply to medical school. The rest is history.

One never knows how a chance interaction is going to change the course of life; but meeting Andy and his family certainly changed mine for the better.

This experience has allowed me to spend the last 26 years of my life devoted to helping others on their health care journey. Thank you, Andy – May God bless you and keep you by His side.

- Dr. Sal

To Andy.

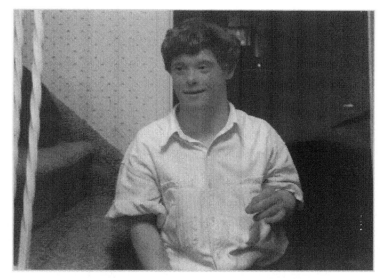

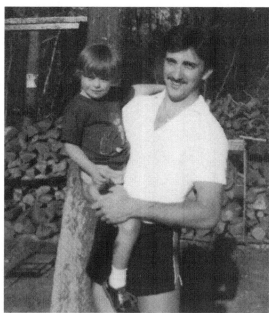

Me with Andy.
Circa 1985

Table of Contents

Preface

This book is a compilation of articles that I have written for *The News-Press*, the *American Journal of Lifestyle Medicine*, and other local and national publications, from October 2015 through December 2019. I have had the pleasure of writing these articles that cover a variety of topics relating to lifestyle behaviors which either promote disease or promote health.

The purpose of each article is to steer the reader on a successful path of health knowing that the six pillars of lifestyle medicine (nutrition, exercise, sleep, stress management, mental well-being, purposeful living) always point us in the right direction. These articles are reader-friendly in length, are easy to read and "get right to the point." They are clear and concise, but will also keep you wanting to learn more. They also help the reader as a student to become the teacher, spreading the message – you CAN grow up and not get OLD!

I hope you enjoy this book. If you feel so inclined, please send comments to drsallifestylemed@gmail.com.

Be Well,
Dr. Sal

Acknowledgement

I'd like to acknowledge my friend, peer and co-champion for health and wellness, Melissa Furman, without whom this book would not have been published.

Melissa worked tirelessly over several months editing and redesigning this book into an enjoyable, readable format.

Melissa was the driving force for the Tulsa VegFest in 2019 and has dedicated much of her life's energy to promoting lifestyle medicine.

She is a wonderful role model for health, wellness and preventive health care and I thank her for being a wonderful part of my life.

-Dr. Sal

Can Gum Disease Lead to Heart Disease?

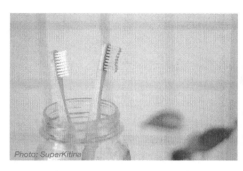

Photo: SuperKitina

During a recent trip to my dentist, it was noticed that I had an area of gum recession and he referred me to a periodontist who agreed with the concern. After a thorough examination, the periodontist recommended a minor surgical procedure to cover the area of recession with a small graft of tissue taken from the top part of the mouth known as the hard palate. When I questioned her on how the gum recession happened, she told me that it could be age related. I laughed and told her she was wrong and there must be another explanation! Even more likely, this was due to overly aggressive brushing (I liked that explanation better). She told me I was brushing incorrectly and actually wearing down the gum around the teeth. As a result, I was increasing the risk for further periodontal disease which in time can increase the risk of heart disease.

Since the association between gum disease and heart disease is not initially obvious, I decided to research this further and write an article which hopefully will help to explain the mechanism. Before I start explaining the mechanism, I will finish the story about the dentist telling me I was not brushing correctly. I thought after 57 years I knew how to brush my teeth! According to the education I got from the dental assistant, I learned how to really clean my teeth using a soft brush (mechanical or manual) and keeping the bristles at an angle so they clean the teeth and do not rub the gums raw. It certainly is important to clean the gums since the mouth is filled with bacteria, yet we do not want to do this so vigorously that we brush the gums away

1

from the teeth. When this occurs, the roots of the teeth are exposed leading to potentially more teeth, gum and bone problems. The bacteria in the mouth, along with food particles and mucus, form a film on the teeth resulting in plaque formation. When plaque is not removed, it eventually becomes tarter which is not removed by brushing. When this occurs, you need to have the tarter professionally removed by the dental hygienist. The longer tarter remains on the teeth the more inflammation it causes. When the gums get inflamed it is called gingivitis. As this process continues, the gums start to pull away from the teeth and form spaces that become infected by bacteria within the mouth. This infection can progress under the gum line and as the immune system tries to fight this infection, toxins are released that break down the connective tissue and the bones holding the teeth in place. Do you see where this is going?

In addition to not brushing properly, there are other risk factors for periodontal disease: smoking, diabetes, hormonal changes and illnesses that affect the immune system, medications which decrease the amount of saliva which helps keep the mouth healthy, other medications which cause an abnormal overgrowth of gum tissue and even genetic susceptibility.

It was interesting for me to see that the gum recession was occurring without symptoms. For other people there might be signs or symptoms including bad breath, red or swollen gums, tender or bleeding gums, painful chewing, sensitive or loose teeth. It is helpful, therefore, to get regular checkups with a dentist to see if there are any signs or symptoms of gum disease or other oral problems. The mouth is also susceptible to cancers; during a screening examination, the dentist will check all areas of the mouth and under the tongue for signs of cancer.

Getting back to the association between periodontal disease and heart disease, how does this happen? If you have read any of my previous articles [in *The News Press*], I explained how inflammation is the common denominator for most chronic illnesses, including gingivitis and periodontitis. When an injury occurs along the gum lining, the immune system becomes activated in order to stop the insult. If the injury or an infection persists, the immune response actually becomes harmful. Bacteria toxins get into the blood stream and activate what is called the systemic immune system. This is the immune system throughout the body. Particles from these bacteria or toxins can get lodged in the heart, liver, kidneys, joints or any other area of the body setting up another immune reaction in these areas. If this continues, the organs themselves become damaged and less functional. Arteriosclerosis (hardening of the arteries) is directly related to inflammation and the more this occurs in the body the more the person is susceptible to heart attacks, strokes and other circulatory problems. Gum disease, therefore, should be added to the list of other risk factors for cardiovascular disease. Since some forms of dementia are related to poor circulation in the brain, gum disease can also be listed as a risk factor for dementia.

In addition to the risk of cardiovascular disease and dementia, gum disease is also associated with diabetes. In this situation, it is the diabetes that increases the risk for the periodontal disease because people with diabetes are more at risk for infections. Nonetheless, the relationship is bi-directional since periodontal disease and persistent inflammation make it harder for the person with diabetes to control their blood sugar. Persistent infections and inflammation cause hormonal changes and continued activation of the immune system, resulting in elevated glucose levels and more complications of uncontrolled diabetes.

As mentioned in previous articles, it all comes down to controlling inflammation. In order to do this we need to know the cause of the inflammation. Once this is ascertained, work can begin on eliminating the cause of the inflammation and decrease the potential complications including gum disease, heart disease, diabetes and dementia.

3

If the periodontist is correct and age is the causative factor for my gum disease, there is not much I can do. If the cause is related to incorrect brushing — self-inflicted injury to the gums — then I can do a lot to make this situation better; I am betting on the latter! Since my visit to the periodontist, I have changed my way of brushing, gotten more diligent with flossing and am now using a water pick to remove the plaque before it becomes tarter. I am focused more now on my teeth in order to keep my heart, brain and other vital organs healthy. In the end I am glad that trip to the dentist resulted in a referral to the periodontist since this might have prevented a future heart attack and saved my brain in the process – thanks to all involved in keeping me healthy!

- Dr. Sal

A Medical Treatment Without Side Effects

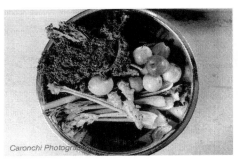

Caronchi Photography

Recently, I had the pleasure of attending a medical conference with 600 other physicians, nutritionists and other health care providers as well as a number of non-medical folks interested in learning how to become and stay healthy. Over a four-day period, we listened to and participated in almost two dozen presentations which all had one central theme - the delivery of a medical treatment with no side effects and only positive benefits.

On Wednesday evening we listened to the keynote speaker, Dr. Kim Williams, the past president of the America College of Cardiology, who espoused the benefits of this blockbuster treatment. On Thursday we heard from the well-known Dr. Dean Ornish who reiterated many of the benefits discussed by Dr. Williams; Dr. Ornish expanded further on this wonder treatment. Dr. Scott Stoll spoke about the central mechanism for most of the chronic illnesses known as inflammation of the arteries and explained how this treatment option represented a cure for most of the medical problems we deal with today. Dr. William Li talked about angiogenesis, the development of new blood vessels; he explained how this medical treatment improved circulation and overall health. Dr. Corey Howard spoke about the microbiome and explained how the bacteria in our GI system is beneficially affected by this medical therapy and how not adopting this medical treatment results in leaky gut syndrome, irritable bowel syndrome and other GI maladies. Dr. Brooke Goldner's talk was about how this medical therapy improves most autoimmune diseases; Dr. Brie Turner-McGrievy spoke about its benefits for women with poly cystic ovarian disease. Dr. Caldwell Esselstyn told us how this treatment option also prevents and reverses cardiovascular disease. He explained in detail how his patients over the last 30 years have been able to reverse the blockages in their arteries and avoid having heart bypass surgery — amazing!

Dr. Craig McDougall told the audience how to implement this wonderful treatment and prevention option in a general medical practice. Next, Micaela Karlsen and Kathy Pollard explained the need for individuals interested in the benefits of this treatment option to commit to changing their behavior if they were to reap its benefits. Lastly, Dr. Michael Greger pulled it all together by talking about hundreds of research studies supporting the benefits of this amazing treatment and prevention option which can benefit everyone on the planet - including those with disease and those without. He reviewed with us many research reports that reinforced the benefits and the reasons why we all should make this prevention and treatment strategy a part of our professional and personal lives.

By now I hope you are sitting on the edge of your seat wondering what this wonder drug is! It is not a drug at all – it is food! Yes, we spent three days hearing about the benefits of food, not just any food - these are plant-based foods. Yes, vegetables! It is amazing to understand how a plant-based nutrition program can prevent disease, treat disease and allow people to live a better quality and a longer life. All of these statements are supported by hundreds, if not thousands, of research studies we heard about during this conference. If you are interested in more details, visit online PlantricianProject.org and NutritionFacts.org. At each of these sites, you can follow links to a significant amount of information that will change your life.

At this point you might be asking, "Why do I need to change my life?" The answer is, because if we don't, then what we have to look forward to as we age is a greater risk of all chronic illnesses and many of the most common cancers. Einstein said the definition of insanity is doing the same thing and expecting a different result. As a nation, if we continue to eat the standard American diet (SAD), the only thing we can count on is the same rates of cardiovascular disease, diabetes, obesity, chronic pain syndromes, autoimmune diseases and cancers.

When we compare longevity for those eating the standard American diet versus those in the world who eat more of a plant-based nutrition program, we see that the populations who eat more vegetables and less meat and dairy live the longest. That is a fact. For the populations who eat more meat and dairy, the risk of more illness is significant; this is one reason I am so passionate about spreading this information to all that are interested.

As I sat and listened to all these wonderful speakers, I kept asking myself, "Why do more people not know about this method of maintaining good health?" Why do we see so many television commercials about medications for heartburn, back pain, high cholesterol and cancer treatment, to name a few? We do not see commercials for healthy eating which we know helps us avoid the diseases these medications are made for. When we treat the cause and not the symptom, we cure and prevent disease. The traditional mentality seems to be: I have a symptom – for example, heartburn - so give me a pill to get rid of the symptom. It would be better to ask, "What is the cause of the symptom and what can I do to eliminate the cause, rather than taking a medication to treat the symptom?" I believe this was the best take-away from the conference I attended. We know that the food we eat creates health or disease. The choices we make at each meal and snack moves us closer to better health or faster into aging and disease.

For 18 years I practiced general internal medicine and it saddened me when patients did not get well. My experience indicated the individuals who took care of themselves by eating healthy food, exercising regularly made health a priority in their lives. Since 2010 when I took the role as the Vice President of Health and Wellness for the Lee Memorial Health System, I have been working diligently with people to prevent disease. My emphasis is finding the cause of the problem rather than simply treating the symptoms. For my patients with high blood pressure, high cholesterol, heart disease, diabetes, obesity and a history of a stroke, I recommend a plant-based nutrition program. For the individuals who are committed to becoming and staying healthy, they transition into this new and healthy lifestyle realizing the benefits over a short period of time.

- Dr. Sal

Is Vitamin D the Only Vitamin Necessary for Strong Bones?

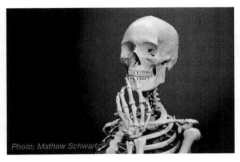

Photo: Mathew Schwartz

Most of us have heard about the importance of Vitamin D in developing and maintaining strong bones yet many have not heard of the importance of Vitamin K for the same purpose. Vitamin D helps put calcium into the bones while Vitamin D without Vitamin K also places calcium into the soft tissues, especially the arteries which then increases the risk for arteriosclerosis (hardening of the arteries).

In actuality, there are two forms of Vitamin K: phylloquinone which is K1 and menaquinone which is K2. Vitamin K1 is involved in blood clotting and K2 is involved in calcification of the bones, preventing calcification of the arteries and produces a protein involved in cell growth regulation (cancer prevention).

Please humor me while I get technical for a few sentences. Chemically, Vitamin K serves as a co-factor for the enzyme GGCX (gamma glutamate carboxylase) which catalyzes the conversion of the amino acid glutamate into Gla (Gammacarboxyglutamate). Basically, this means that Vitamin K is necessary for specific chemical reactions to occur in order for the body to produce several different proteins. This helps us understand that a vitamin is simply a substance that the body needs to allow a chemical reaction to occur.

Gla is responsible for the production of several proteins including Osteocalcin (a protein needed for bone formation), MGP a matrix Gla protein (which prevents calcification of the arteries) and Gas6 (growth arrest sequence protein) which is the protein involved in

9

cell growth regulation. The proteins involved in blood clotting are produced in the liver. The other proteins mentioned are produced in various organs such as the bones and arteries. From a life sustaining perspective, the work that goes on in the liver to ensure the production of clotting takes precedence over the production of other proteins.

Vitamin K1 makes up 90% of the Vitamin K found in the western diet and is found in green leafy vegetables such as spinach, Swiss chard, parsley, as well as kale, broccoli and Brussels sprouts. It is also found in avocado, kiwi and grapes.

Vitamin K2 is found in the Japanese food called natto (fermented soybean) as well as some fermented cheese and curds. Bacteria involved in the fermentation actually produce the vitamin. Intestinal uptake of Vitamin K is affected by the foods we eat and uptake appears to be increased when Vitamin K foods are eaten with fats. Once absorbed, all K vitamins are transported to the liver where they are used for the production of blood clotting factors. Once this function is satisfied, K2 is then transported to the bones and arteries for the production of the other proteins mentioned above.

Since the body has this built-in mechanism to ensure the production of clotting factors, vitamin K1 deficiency is not usually a problem; when deficiency of Vitamin K2 occurs, it can appear as problems in the bones and arteries.

Over the past fifty years, food sources in the U.S. have been produced with less Vitamin K; therefore, more people are becoming K deficient. One reason is that cows are now fed grain rather than grass; and, cows that eat corn do not produce vitamin K2 rich milk. The end result of vitamin deficient food are weak bones that are more susceptible to osteoporosis and fractures; and, arteries that have more calcium in the walls make them stiffer and more prone to arteriosclerosis (hardening of the arteries).

When it comes to vitamin levels, there is a difference between a true deficiency and an insufficiency. True Vitamin K deficiency would produce serious bleeding problems. Vitamin D deficiency produces a disease called rickets and Vitamin C deficiency produces scurvy. The Recommended Daily Allowances (RDA) for vitamins have been defined to prevent true deficiencies. What happens when a person develops an insufficient vitamin level? Prolonged vitamin insufficiency results in what we consider age-related illnesses; namely, osteoporosis and arteriosclerosis. Vitamin C is an anti-oxidant, so when the level is low (insufficient but not deficient), the body is more susceptible to oxidation (rusting from within). When Vitamin D is low, there is an increased risk for a number of diseases including cancer and some neuromuscular diseases such as multiple sclerosis. When Vitamin K2 is not sufficient, there is an increased risk for cancer and other illnesses as mentioned.

Since it appears that Vitamin K insufficiency is increasing as the quality of the food in the U.S. declines, increasing the dietary intake of Vitamin K might be important in improving the health of the general population. For children, this is vital since the requirement for the Vitamin K dependent protein called Osteocalcin (needed for bone development) is much higher than for adults. In older adults, the lack of Vitamin K results in what has been termed age-related diseases. As we see from the explanation above, osteoporosis and arteriosclerosis are at least partially related to Vitamin D and K insufficiency. These disorders probably occur because of multiple reasons; hence, getting rid of one risk factor may contribute substantially to postponing the disease.

For people with Crohn's disease and cystic fibrosis, impaired intestinal absorption results in multiple vitamin deficiencies; therefore, supplementation is beneficial. It is known that Vitamin K supplementation is beneficial and safe; the exception is a person taking a blood thinner (such as Warfarin or Coumadin), as supplemental Vitamin K will interfere with the effects of this medication. Physicians usually recommend staying away from supplemental Vitamin K when taking blood thinners. In these situations, it is important to check the level of vitamin K in the blood to be sure insufficiency or deficiency are not occurring, increasing the risk for bone loss and hardening of the arteries.

In summary, we can now understand the importance of Vitamin K as well as Vitamin D in the prevention of osteoporosis, arterial calcification, the development of arteriosclerosis and even in the production of cancer. In my previous News-Press articles, I have explained the widespread benefits of Vitamin D and we now see Vitamin K also has a multitude of beneficial effects in addition to the production of blood clotting factors. Since the best source of most vitamins is food, we again see the benefits of healthy eating. The best way to become and stay healthy is through healthy eating. By eating real foods, foods grown and not processed in a chemistry lab, we are able to maintain optimal health with emphasis on the word **optimal**. Our health goal should be for optimal health, not just the absence of disease. Optimal health allows us to be energetic, vital and maximally functional. It enables us to age gracefully and fitfully. Good health lets us wake up looking forward to another day without illness, medication and doctor visits. So eat well, take your vitamins, be active mentally and physically and stay well, my friends.

- Dr. Sal

How Important is Postmenopausal Estrogen Replacement?

Estrogen hormone replacement is only important if you are concerned about healthy aging. It is really important to every woman interested in living a long and fulfilling life! Now that I have your attention, let's review some facts about estrogen.

We know that estrogen has beneficial effects on the brain, heart, vascular system, blood pressure, mood, the immune system and many other functions. A recent article in Frontiers in Physiology questioned if estrogen is the fountain of youth. This article appeared in the June 2012 edition, volume 3, article #165, for those interested in reading it. The focus was on the vascular changes that occur with aging and specifically, looking at risk factors for cardiovascular disease in women as they age. It explains in great detail the importance of maintaining an optimal level of estrogen and what happens when a woman is deficient. Replacement of estrogen in postmenopausal women has significant benefits including effects on the blood vessels, the immune system and the nervous system in the brain. In the blood vessels, estrogen increases the production of nitric oxide, one of the most important chemicals involved in dilating blood vessels. Estrogen decreases inflammation in the blood vessels, helps decrease the level of oxygen radicals, substances within the blood that cause the cells to rust, influences the metabolism of lipids and other hormones, relaxes the blood vessels, decreases blood pressure and reduces the development of arteriosclerosis referred to as hardening of the arteries.

When estrogen levels start to decline, the woman may experience hot flashes, night sweats, vaginal dryness, anxiety, mood swings, depression, insomnia, weight gain and bloating. Estrogen

13

deficiency increases the risk for cardiovascular diseases (heart attacks, strokes and high blood pressure), cognitive decline and dementia, psychiatric and psychological problems and more. In reviewing the literature for this article, I found a citation which stated that estrogen has 400 functions within the body. No wonder so many problems can occur when this hormone declines! Estrogen also has effects on glucose metabolism and the body's response to insulin. It helps maintain a normal metabolic rate and influences the level of thyroid hormone. It also affects sleep and overall stress levels.

When we start to discuss estrogen replacement therapy (ERT), we have to review the details regarding synthetic versus bio-identical hormones. Synthetic estrogen is not the same as estrogen made naturally. The most commonly used synthetic estrogen comes from the urine of pregnant mares and contains many different forms of estrogen. In comparison, bio-identical estrogen is the same as what is made naturally by a woman's ovaries. The goal is to replace estrogen with the most natural form and in a form most helpful to the woman as she ages. Most of the bio-identical forms of estrogen contain estradiol and estriol, aka E2 and E3, respectively.

In the body, estrogen is metabolized to other substances, some which are healthful and some increase a woman's risk of disease, including cancer. The goal, therefore, is to increase the body's ability to metabolize estrogen into the more healthful versions; this can be done with supplements including B vitamins (B2, B6 and B12), folic acid, eating cruciferous vegetables (broccoli and cauliflower), freshly ground flax seeds and soy products. It also helps to include Omega 3 fatty acids (fish oil), turmeric, rosemary and plant protein in meals. Of course, don't forget the importance of exercise and stress reduction!

There are situations where metabolism goes in the wrong direction and this occurs when the woman is overweight, has a low thyroid level, exposed to pesticides and other environmental chemicals; and, when the body is more inflamed. There are over 50 environmental chemicals known to negatively affect estrogen. These are known as Xenoestrogens; and, in addition to pesticides, include estrogens fed to animals as well as synthetic estrogens found in plastics and cosmetics.

The effects of animal products (meat and dairy) on estrogen metabolism are significant and should be clearly understood in order for every individual to make decisions for him/her regarding nutrition. In addition to the artificial estrogen that comes along with the steak and cheese in the standard American diet, the antibiotics that are fed to the cattle, pigs and chickens also influence the natural estrogen balance. These antibiotics affect the normal bacteria in a person's GI tract, called the microbiome, and the normal metabolism of estrogen. There have been research reports describing an increased risk of breast and prostate cancer in such situations. Yes, estrogen is also important to men.

Estrogen also has significant effects on the brain such as increasing blood flow, oxygen and glucose levels, protecting the nerve cells, increasing the levels of neurotransmitters (chemicals needed for brain cell communication), decreasing the production of amyloid proteins which cause dementia and stabilizing the blood-brain barrier.

How is the estrogen level measured? Should a woman also be checked for the level of estrogen metabolites? Estrogen levels can be tested from blood, saliva and urine samples. Blood tests will give information about the current levels of E1, E2 and E3. Saliva testing is useful to get a full 24-hour perspective and the urine test is good to look at the metabolites of estrogen.

The processes involved in estrogen production, metabolism and degradation require many different enzymes as well as normal liver function. If the levels of necessary enzymes are not adequate, then either the metabolism or the breakdown is affected leading to the accumulation of toxic substances. This is where healthy nutrition comes into the equation. We all need to supply the body with the proper amounts of healthy proteins, fats, carbohydrates, vitamins, mineral and antioxidants. Proteins, fats and carbohydrates are the macro nutrients the body requires to rebuild and repair itself. The micronutrients are the vitamins, minerals and antioxidants which the body needs for all the chemical reactions described earlier to occur. This pertains to the chemical reactions that allow us to use food to make energy, produce new cells, repair damage, fight infection and destroy cancer cells.

Overall health requires not only hormone replacement, which should be balanced to optimal levels; it also requires adequate amounts of healthy food and drink. The standard American diet includes an overwhelming amount of unhealthy fats, sugar, salt and contaminants all of which effect the hormone balance but more importantly, leads us down the road to chronic illness, cancer and a shortened life. I use the word optimal intentionally. My idea of good health is optimal health, not just health at a level that allows us to avoid disease. Lack of disease is not optimal health. So…let's shoot for the stars! Balance estrogen and other hormones to optimal levels, eat the healthiest food you can find (invest in your health), stay active physically and mentally; live life to the fullest!

- Dr. Sal

Protein – What's All the Chatter About?

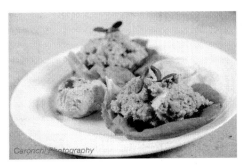

Caronchi Photography

We hear and read so much these days about the need for dietary protein but what is all the hype about? Certainly, protein is important. The origin of the word even tells us that it is primary, meaning we must pay attention to it! As a macronutrient, protein is certainly primary, along with fats and carbohydrates. You cannot live without all the major macronutrients. The same goes for the micronutrients that will be discussed below.

A lot of what is written about protein has to do with how much we should consume and whether we should be eating animal versus plant protein; and, if we take in more plant protein, are we able to get enough protein to support our bodily functions?

Let's start by discussing the functions of the macronutrients. Proteins are needed to build skeletal muscles, for synthesis of hormones and other vital chemicals, to make up cell structures and other physical parts of the body. Fats are necessary for the composition of the brain, nervous system, cell membranes, as well as contributing to the production of cholesterol, bile and other chemical compounds. Carbohydrates are a needed source of fuel, as are fats, and for the production of hormones and enzymes that are needed for the millions of chemical reactions occurring in the body daily. All three are needed on a daily basis and diets that intentionally omit one of these essential macronutrients are not completely healthy.

Micronutrients are the vitamins, antioxidants and minerals that are essential for health. These are enzymes and other co-factors which participate in chemical reactions such as digestion, absorption of nutrients, production of hormones, synthesis of proteins, detoxification, repair and rebuilding of injured cells and tissues. They are not substitutes for macronutrients or food. You cannot skip a meal, take a vitamin and think you will stay healthy. The vitamins and minerals are needed for the body to use the proteins, fats and carbohydrates that you eat. The body is one big chemical factory needing the right ingredients to function efficiently.

Now that we know why we need all these elements, let's discuss the need for protein and which type might be healthier. Animal versus plant protein -- there are pros and cons for each. Animal protein is a more complete protein, yet it comes with a price. We need to think about animal protein (meat and dairy) as <u>processed food</u>, understanding the reality of what happens to the animals before they are slaughtered (one billion annually in the U.S. alone!). Because the producers (no longer called farmers) want to get these animals big and fat and ready for slaughter as fast as possible, they give them antibiotics and hormones to accelerate their growth. This is an unnatural process for the animals, contributing to suffering. In addition to adding muscle mass, these animals also add fat and this, in addition to the antibiotics and hormones, contributes to the unhealthiness of this protein source. In addition, processed animal protein (red meat, chicken, pork and lunch meat) is often contaminated with fecal material and bacteria, as well as pesticides from the grain they eat. The grain fed to these animals does not allow them to develop the same amount of healthy omega 3 fatty acids that they would normally, if they were eating grass. The meat is not as healthy as compared to animals raised on a traditional farm grazing on grass.

We can still compare the biological value of animal protein to that of plant protein to see the scale tip in favor of animal protein as per the strict definition. The quality of a protein is measured as its BV, or biological value. Another measure is called the protein equivalent ratio (PER) and another is called the PDCAA score (the protein digestibility corrected amino acid score). No matter what quality indicator you use, the animal protein comes up higher. As mentioned above, the animal protein comes with a lot of contamination that is known to cause most of the common chronic illnesses and many of the cancers. A great source for this information is in *The China Study* by T. Colin Campbell. Since cardiovascular disease and cancers are the number one and two killers of people in the U.S. and most developed countries, we need to pay close attention to these facts. Researchers continue working to cure these health problems - how about preventing them in the first place? There are thousands of research reports supporting the relationship between better health and less animal products. As a society, we must start to pay attention to these facts. We as a nation have become unhealthier over the last 50 years and we are raising a generation of children thought to have a shorter life expectancy than their parents. What a horrible thought!

Let's look at the alternative – plant/vegetable protein. When we look at the measures of plant protein quality (the BV, PER or PDCAA score), we see lower numbers. An egg is considered the standard for animal protein with a score of 1.0 meaning that the body is able to use all of this protein even though it comes with much contamination. In comparison, kidney beans have a score of 0.68, lentils 0.52 and soy protein 0.47. When we factor in the contamination of animal products, we get the feeling that plant sources of protein lead to better health and this is exactly what the research shows. Yes, we know that many vegetables are contaminated with pesticides, especially when they are genetically modified. This is one reason to buy organic produce. Fruits or vegetables with a thin skin should be organic. Look online for the **dirty dozen** and make sure you buy these foods as organic. The labels on the produce should start with the number nine – this is how you know it is organic. If the label starts with the number four, it is conventionally grown and exposed to

19

pesticides; and, if it starts with the number eight, it is genetically modified. GMOs are food products that have had their DNA modified to better resist pesticides and herbicides causing more contamination. Apparently, the majority of corn and soy produced in the U.S. are genetically modified; therefore, it is most important to buy only non-GMO corn and soy products.

When discussing this topic with folks, I find many eating the Paleo diet. This refers to how people in the Paleolithic era fed themselves. For many, it seems as if they use this method to justify eating more meat; in reality, humans living in Paleolithic times ate less meat, since they had to hunt and kill the animals they wanted to eat. Can you see today's humans doing this? In contrast, we prefer the fast food drive through line to get our meat! This type of eating is more in line with the Atkins diet, which allows most of the calories to come from animal products (meat and dairy). If you prefer and feel better eating meat, then buy organic, grass fed, farm raised antibiotic and hormone-free meat. You can order these types of meat online or buy them in some of the better grocery stores. Do this in moderation because even though these animals are raised differently, the meat and dairy still come with a lot of unhealthy fat which contributes to the cardiovascular disease and cancer that many of our family members and friends deal with every day. Again, let's focus on prevention as opposed to a cure! Please forget the lunch meat since these animal products contain nitrites, which are more associated with cancer than traditional meat and dairy. Sorry, I am just the deliverer of the message and I do this because my passion is to help people stay healthy!

If you decide to eat less animal protein and more plant/vegetable protein, how much do you need? Most people who have this conversation with me ask, "How will I get enough protein if I don't eat meat?" The answer is you will get enough if you eat many different types of vegetables along with legumes, seeds and nuts. Actually, when you compare the same number of calories of meat protein versus plant protein, you get healthier protein from the plants since the meat comes with a lot of fat calories and less protein calories. Also, with vegetables you do not have to worry about counting calories because vegetables are nutrient dense which means more nutrients with fewer calories – so eat as much as you want. Your weight will be healthier, and you might actually feel better! When we look at the actual amount of protein grams required, it is generally about 1 gram per kilogram which means for an average 70 kg man (150 lbs), he would need 70 grams per day. Women require less, and athletes require more. The standard egg contains about 5 grams of protein. Two cups of broccoli have about the same. Most plant-based protein powders used to make a smoothie contains 20 grams. One cup of kidney beans contains almost 8 grams. A four-ounce steak contains about 30 grams. Two cups of kale equal 5 grams. All of this information is easily accessible online, or if you use a smart phone, just ask Siri.

It is important to look beyond the numbers in order to determine the healthiest source of protein; and, when factoring in all the contaminants that come with so many of the foods we eat and drink, we must consider the effects these contaminants have on us. In addition to what has been mentioned above, there are many different chemicals in various food and drink products. For example, these include food additives such as colorings, flavorings and preservatives. These are all toxins to the natural chemistry of the body. They affect the ability of the mitochondria to make energy, shorten the ends of the DNA telomeres and speed up the aging process. They strain the liver and the body's detoxification system, increase the risk of Alzheimer's, endothelial dysfunction and many other chronic illnesses and cancer. The body craves healthy, nutritious, non-contaminated food and drink. When we eat foods laden with toxins, unhealthy fats, disease producing amounts of sugar and salt, we decrease the quality of our lives and shorten our lifespan - that's a fact!

Staying healthy requires intentional thought and energy when deciding each meal and snack. Meal planning is essential if you want to stay healthy and avoid disease. Before you go shopping, make a detailed list of the healthy items you want to buy; for example, organic spinach, broccoli, fruits, almond milk and, if you prefer, non-dairy cheese. If you are set on eating meat, avoid lunch meat and instead get farm raised, organic, antibiotic and hormone free, grass-fed meat and limit this to no more than four ounces a few times per week. Add a salad to lunch and dinner meals, eat a handful of nuts and seeds for healthy fats. Drink lots of water -- at least 48 oz. per day assuming no heart or kidney problems; and, get lots of fiber in the diet to keep the GI tract moving.

If you think you need to take vitamins, have a micronutrient blood test to see if you are deficient in any of the essential vitamins, minerals or antioxidants. It is better to be academic about your supplements, so you do not expose yourself to unnecessary risk by taking too many supplements. This way is less expensive.

Avoid sugar as much as you can, since glucose and other sugar molecules such as fructose attach to all proteins causing the development of advanced glycation end products also known as AGEs. When sugar attaches to proteins in the body, the proteins are not able to function normally; this leads to a host of illnesses including vascular disease, Alzheimer's and other degenerative diseases.

If you are concerned about getting enough protein, you must be concerned about getting enough sleep. In order to use the protein to build skeletal muscle, you need to make growth hormone, and this is made at night during restful sleep. By getting enough sleep, you make the GH necessary to build healthy skeletal muscle; and, this is where many calories are burned allowing you to maintain a healthy metabolism as well as an ideal body weight.

In addition, keep the stress level down since high stress for long periods of time increases cortisol and increases weight. It increases the fat accumulation under the skin and even more detrimentally around the vital organs such as the heart, kidney and

22

liver. Fat also increases inflammation in the body and this increases the risk for all chronic illnesses, cancer and even dementia.

With the right amount of protein, you can **schedule the exercise** you need to stay healthy. The more intensely you exercise, the more fat you burn. Include strength training in your exercise routine since this will help keep insulin and other hormones in balance. It is recommended that you talk with your physician or health care provider before starting any exercise program. Also, talk with your exercise specialist about post-exercise protein meals which are needed to repair the minor muscle damage caused by exercise. Exercise is necessary for the muscles, bones and the rest of the body to stay healthy and to decrease the aging process. A post-exercise protein meal allows for quicker recovery between exercise sessions.

Another great book to read as an educational resource to help you understand the topics described above is called *Rethink Foods* by Amy Goodman. Other authors include Dr. Michael Greger, Dr. Joel Fuhrman and Dr. Neal Barnard. Go online to www.Nutritonfacts.org to listen to Dr. Greger's daily messages about nutrition.

- Dr. Sal

What Does the Bathroom Scale Reveal About Your Health?

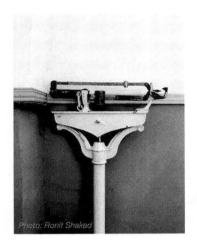

Photo: Ronit Shaked

Traditional bathroom scales measure weight alone; we can now invest in a higher-grade scale which calculates body fat percent as well as body mass index (BMI). Are these more expensive scales worth the additional money and what are the reasons we need to know these additional numbers?

First, let's look at weight alone to consider what it tells us about health. Body weight is a measure of the combined weight of a person's bones, muscles, fat and organs. It allows us to compare one person's weight to another person of similar height and from this to calculate a BMI. The body mass index is a comparison of a person's weight versus their height; telling something about their overall health. If a person is 5'4" tall and weighs 250 lbs., he/she is significantly overweight; if the person is 6'4" tall and also weighs 250 lbs., the weight is not as much of an issue.

By looking at the other measurements which can be obtained from more advanced scales, the percentage of body fat is a very useful measurement since this differentiates fat weight from the weight attributable to bone and muscle. This is an important detail because the more fat we accumulate under the skin, the more at risk we are for diabetes, metabolic syndrome, cardiovascular disease, dementia, cancers, musculoskeletal disorders and depression. Fat accumulates not only under the skin but detrimentally around all the vital organs such as the heart, kidneys and liver. This is termed visceral fat or

24

organ fat; and, the reason this is so dangerous is because it interferes with the function of these vital organs. As weight increases, so does the risk for heart related problems, kidney disease and liver dysfunction. The long-term consequences of visceral fat include slowly progressive failure of these organs. The heart may become enlarged and dysfunctional. The kidneys and liver are no longer able to function efficiently. A disorder called non-alcoholic fatty liver disease (NAFLD) increases the risk for cirrhosis and liver cancer. With this explanation, you can understand the relationship between being overweight and having an increased risk for cancer.

As fat accumulates, it surrounds the organs and also accumulates under the skin – this is called subcutaneous fat (SQ). This is also a health risk since fat cells are not just passively sitting under the skin (or around the organs). Fat cells produce chemicals and hormones which cause inflammation throughout the entire body. If you have been reading my previous News-Press articles, inflammation is the root cause of most of the chronic illnesses and many of the most common cancers people suffer with today. Inflammation increases the risk for Alzheimer's dementia, cardiovascular diseases, many autoimmune and musculoskeletal disorders, diabetes and metabolic syndrome.

The accumulation of subcutaneous and visceral fat is therefore a significant present and long-term health risk. If you do not have a fancy scale to take these measurements, there is another way to get this information. One way to get an indication of the risks is to calculate a waist-to-hip ratio. Simply measure your waist at the level of the belly button and hip circumference at the level of the top of the femur (the big bone at the top of the leg) and calculate the ratio. The higher the ratio is, the more at risk you are. As the belly gets bigger, so does the health risk. As the hips get bigger so does the health risk. Men accumulate much of the fat in their abdomen (referred to as a beer belly). Women accumulate fat around the hips and buttocks making them more pear-shaped. In either situation, the result is the same. The more SQ fat, the more visceral fat and the more health problems occur.

As I roam around the neighborhood, I am sad to see how many young children have beer bellies and pear-shaped bodies. It is important for parents to understand this is not healthy and in the long run significantly increases the child's risk for all the medical problems cited above. Parents of an overweight child have the responsibility to set a good health example for their children and also need to develop a defined action plan for an overweight child to lose weight and get healthier.

Let's discuss how we can have a significant impact on the problem of obesity among people of all ages in the U.S. today. Initially, we must accept this as a problem and plan to be active in the solution. I suggest parents use a small index card and write on it: "help (name of child) get healthier"; or, for the adolescent or adult with a weight problem, write on the card something like "focus on a healthier weight." Take the card out of your pocket many times during the day and read the words. Then ask yourself if you are doing all you can on that day to achieve this goal. I make this suggestion because focusing on a goal and thinking about it often gets us closer to achieving it.

Next, I would suggest meeting with a nutritionist who can help make sense out of what you or your children are currently eating and offer suggestions for improvement. The standard American way of eating more processed foods, high sugar drinks, animal products loaded with fat as well as many other contaminants, junk food, etc., has over the past 50 years led Americans down the road to many of the health problems detailed above. Since we know the problems, let's work to create a palatable solution! One way to do this is to slowly introduce healthier foods and drinks into each meal. I emphasize the slow approach since it takes time to enjoy foods that you have never eaten before; once you start to see how many great, delicious foods you have been missing out on, you will wonder why you did not begin sooner!

As part of the solution, I recommend to all my patients meal planning and for those working, bringing lunch to work. Buy a decent-sized cooler and fill it with a healthy salad, pre-cut vegetables, a few fruits or healthy snacks that will get you through the day. Drink water with each meal and avoid soda. Did you know that one soda daily for one year can add 13 lbs. to the hips?

Many of my patients have been through the CHIP (Complete Health Improvement Program) which teaches people how to shop for, cook and enjoy many foods not found in the standard American diet. In nine weeks the average person loses 10-12 lbs.; more importantly, many of these folks get off medications for high blood pressure, diabetes, and a slew of other medical problems. They all talk about how much better they feel with more energy and mental clarity. After the program ends, they have more time to ramp up the exercise adding even more to the health gains achieved. It is amazing to see how focusing on what we eat and how much we move and exercise, make such a difference in our overall present and future health.

As we progress along this road toward better health, we can periodically go back to the scale and compare the changes in weight and body fat percentage. The goal is to lose fat and gain muscle since muscle burns more calories than fat cells do. When developing an exercise routine, make sure to do some weight lifting. Weight lifting adds muscle and strengthens the bones, thereby increasing the metabolic rate and decreasing the risk for osteoporosis. This is a win-win all the way around!

If you don't want to buy a new scale, you can come to the Wellness Center where I work and have these measurements done on the Tanita scale that I use for the folks I work with. Once you know your numbers, you can make a plan as suggested above to decrease the weight, get rid of some of that harmful fat, build healthier muscles and bones, increase your metabolism and get yourself healthier!

Remember, we only get one shot at this life and it is urgent to get healthier as fast as possible since none of us know how long we have on this great planet!

- Dr. Sal

Stress, Health and the Adrenal Glands

In this fast paced world we live in today, many people complain of fatigue. When I see these folks in the office, I have to think about the many different medical problems that might be causing the fatigue including anemia, low thyroid, depression, poor nutrition, fibromyalgia, medication side effects, lack of sleep and too much stress, to name a few.

In relation to excessive stress, we have to consider what is termed adrenal fatigue. There are several severe problems that can occur with the adrenal glands ranging from significantly low function (Addison's disease) to hyper-function (Cushing's disease/syndrome). These are much less common than the condition in the mid-range known as adrenal fatigue. When people live under conditions of chronic stress, over time the adrenal glands will burn out. The adrenal glands secrete cortisol allowing a person to deal with acute stress effectively. If the stress continues, the glands begin to fail, and the person starts to develop signs and symptoms consistent with low cortisol. The health consequences include an increased risk for asthma, allergies, autoimmune diseases and cancers. The immune function is compromised, the heart cannot pump effectively, and the person complains of low energy and no stamina. The individual has a difficult time getting through the work day and requires frequent naps, yet still does not feel rested.

When the physician looks at the function of the adrenal gland using typical blood tests, he/she sees a pattern of cortisol fluctuations that is different from other fatigue syndromes; and, this is consistent with the person's energy pattern throughout the day. The physician questions the individual about their life and realizes there is constant

29

stress which may be work related, due to difficult relationships, or emotional stress from a recent divorce or death. When the discussion turns to the person's eating habits, it becomes clear that the person has certain food cravings (salty and fatty foods) as well as other food intolerances, such as not being able to tolerate carbohydrates without eating fats or proteins at the same time. Blood testing will reveal hypoglycemia (low blood sugar) especially after a carbohydrate meal. The physical examination will often reveal low-blood pressure especially when the person goes from lying or sitting to standing - they feel lightheaded.

One of the best tests to diagnose adrenal fatigue is a salivary cortisol test done at four different times in a 24-hour period. Another good blood test is called a glucose tolerance test which reveals if the person has difficulty handling a sugar load, causing fluctuations in insulin and glucose making the person jittery and lightheaded due to hypoglycemia.

In addition to looking at the cortisol level, the physician/health care provider can also look at the hormones that control the release of cortisol from the adrenals including adrenocorticotropin hormone (ACTH) which comes from the pituitary gland; and, corticotrophin releasing hormone (CRH) from the area of the brain called the hypothalamus. These hormones represent the hypothalamic-pituitary-adrenal (HPA) axis which is a complex hormone system that helps keep all these hormones in balance; and, helps keep the person maximally healthy.

The many different hormones in the body are working in symphony; therefore, in addition to measuring the cortisol level, the physician will also measure other hormones including thyroid, progesterone, estrogen, testosterone and DHEA.

Hypothyroid, described as low thyroid function, is another common reason for chronic fatigue. This should be ruled out as part of the workup for adrenal fatigue. It is important to understand that cortisol is necessary to maintain normal thyroid hormone levels since cortisol functions at three different areas relating to the thyroid hormone. Cortisol is required for the release to TSH, the controlling hormone from the pituitary. It is also required for the liver to convert T4 into the active thyroid hormone, T3; cortisol is also necessary at the receptor sites where thyroid hormone has its action on the cells.

In order to be optimally healthy, all hormone levels must be in balance; therefore, looking at the symphony and balancing all the hormones which are not in an optimal range is necessary. I use the word **optimal** specifically since the goal is to replace hormones to a level where the person is optimally healthy and not simply to a level where the person is not at risk for a disease. Being truly healthy means being optimally functional; and, the lack of disease is not the definition of true health.

What can be done once a person is diagnosed with adrenal fatigue? As with so many other illnesses, lifestyle changes make such a difference. The individual is given recommendations on nutrition, exercise, stress management and sleep. If needed, there is a discussion about supplements realizing it is most important to get the needed vitamins, minerals and antioxidants from healthy food and drink. As with the hormone levels, the physician can also measure the levels of all vitamins, minerals and anti- oxidants; if low, they can be supplemented. Important supplements include vitamin C, B-complex vitamins including niacin and B6; biotin, calcium, magnesium and other trace elements.

In addition, there are other herbal remedies called adaptogens that balance the adrenal glands. These herbal remedies will be recommended by integrative medicine or naturopathic medicine physicians and have been shown in many clinical studies to be very effective. Adding these to mainstream medical treatment for low adrenal function, provides a more comprehensive treatment plan.

In closing, let me emphasize the importance of stress management since this is the causitive factor for adrenal fatigue in the first place - prevention is the best cure! Thus, it is important to look at the reasons why stress is occurring and make a defined action plan to decrease some of the stress. This might sound impossible to do at first; yet, if this is not done, the adrenal function will continue to decline and overall health fades away. Disease occurs forcing a person to make lifestyle changes. It is best to <u>make voluntary changes</u> to decrease stress before life dictates involuntary changes. Do all you can each day to safeguard your health, avoid disease and disability.

- Dr. Sal

Do You Know Your Stress Hormone Level?

When we think about health, how much emphasis do we place on decreasing the stress level in our daily lives? How does stress effect health in the short and long term? Stress is a double-edged sword. During an acutely stressful event, such as being chased by a dog, the stress reaction releases adrenalin, cortisol and other hormones allow you to use your muscles to run away; and, the reaction supplies your muscles with glucose and fatty acids as an energy source. This reaction stimulates your heart to pump more frequently and vigorously, while raising the blood pressure as part of this fight-or-flight response. Blood is shunted away from the intestines. You do not need to worry about digesting food when you are running away from danger or you might end up being the food! Preferentially, the body shunts blood to the heart and skeletal muscles, so they may work overtime. These reactions represent a survival mechanism; and, once the threat is gone, these hormone levels return to normal, the pulse and blood pressure come down and the systems return to a de-stressed condition.

When stress is prolonged, the changes that occur in the various hormones and chemicals within the body and brain become harmful and can be potentially life threatening. Chronic stress occurs for many reasons such as bad relationships at home, excessive and prolonged stress at work, illness, death of a loved one, divorce, excessive extreme exercise and poor nutrition. During these situations the body continues to release cortisol, the stress hormone; other hormones are also involved such as adrenalin, thyroid hormone (for metabolism), melatonin (for sleep) and the sex hormones estrogen, progesterone and testosterone. Stress affects not only cortisol but many of the other hormones in the symphony. I have used the word *symphony* in previous articles since hormones play together in concert and must all be in balance for the person to be optimally healthy.

What are the signs and symptoms of cortisol excess? Glucose (sugar) levels in the body are elevated as well as the lipids (cholesterol). Blood pressure is higher than normal; and, the body's ability to deal with infection decreases since immunity is impaired. Over time we see a redistribution of fat around the face and abdomen; and, underneath the skin, fat accumulates around the vital organs impairing their function. The red blood cell levels elevate increasing the risk for blood clots while the white blood cell levels decline increasing the risk for infection. In the brain, excess cortisol affects the hippocampus which is the memory center, thereby increasing the risk for dementia as well as depression.

If stress persists for a prolonged period, the adrenal gland responses start to fail, and this is when adrenal fatigue becomes obvious. The levels of cortisol start to fall and we then see signs and symptoms of a decrease in cortisol including low blood sugar, low blood pressure, reduced stores of fat as well as skeletal muscle; and, an increased risk for autoimmune disorders, those conditions where the body produces antibodies that attack itself. The individual in this situation often presents to the doctor complaining of fatigue, decreased motivation, difficulty getting out of bed in the morning, depression, unintentional weight loss, decreased strength and loss of libido.

There are many reasons for fatigue including anemia, low thyroid, depression, chronic infection, cancer, side effects of medications, low blood pressure, unbalanced hormones, poor nutrition/vitamin deficiency and impaired heart function to name a few. It is most important, therefore, to see your physician/health care provider if symptoms persist. A workup will include a complete physical examination, blood tests and a comprehensive history of lifestyle behaviors and social issues. This allows your physician to focus on problem areas of the body and the brain. Once this is known, an appropriate treatment plan can be developed. A plan for recurrence, what I call a prevention plan, should also be formed.

In addition to the above, we have been learning about the connection between stress and GI function. The gastrointestinal system which includes the stomach, intestines, gallbladder, liver and pancreas is tremendously influenced by stress. This is one reason people get ulcers, irritable bowel disorder and leaky gut. Even more importantly, we now know chronic stress damages the lining of the GI tract, allowing toxins to get into the blood stream inflicting damage to many areas of the body and brain.

Even more concerning, chronic stress has been shown to increase the aging process by damaging the ends of the chromosomes (telomeres) as well as the mitochondria (the energy powerhouse of all cells). Chronic stress shortens the telomeres advancing the aging process; and, damage to the mitochondria decreases the cells' ability to make energy.

How do we check the stress hormone level? This can be done by measuring the level of cortisol in the blood, urine or saliva. The goal is to measure levels at various times of the day knowing that cortisol levels fluctuate throughout the day naturally in response to stress and other life events. When we know what is happening to the cortisol levels over the 24-hour period, we can then work on a treatment plan.

The first part of the treatment plan must involve identifying the cause of the stress; and, we need to work to eliminate as much of this as possible. If this is done and the adrenals are still not functioning, normally your physician can give supplemental cortisone and can replace other deficient hormones. The tests for cortisol will usually be accompanied by tests for several other hormones including thyroid and the sex hormones, estrogen, progesterone and testosterone. Again, it is most important to balance the symphony of hormones. In addition to replacing deficient hormones, the treatment plan will include optimizing nutrition, adding Adaptogens to the plan, and developing a stress management, sleep and exercise program. Adaptogens are herbs and other supplements (usually given by an integrative medicine or naturopathic physician) which help balance the adrenal glands.

In summary, it is apparent we must intentionally look at the level of stress in our lives, measure the stress hormone cortisol as well as other hormones mentioned above; then decrease the cause of the stress as much as possible to support the adrenal glands as they heal and get back to normal function. This may take sometime; yet, with proper management as described above, the adrenal function usually gets back to normal and life is good again!

- Dr. Sal

Health Requires a Change in Mindset

Recently I had the extreme pleasure of listening to Dr. David Perlmutter discuss the microbiome, a topic I have written about several times in the News-Press. He opened the presentation with a picture of what looked like a parrot and stated we need to start looking at the world differently and thinking differently. He then revealed the picture of a parrot was actually a painted lady. It was a fantastic visual to go along with his opening statement!

From the start of his presentation, I was on the edge of my seat since I have been on my own journey. When it comes to the causes of disease and our ability to become and stay healthy, we need to look at the world differently. I would like to engage the reader to think about the myriad of chronic illnesses and cancers so many people in America are plagued with and ask why. Why is it that so many people in the developed countries come down with heart disease, diabetes, dementia, irritable bowel syndrome, chronic pain syndromes, cancer and depression? Why is it that we see so many children with autism, attention deficit disorder and asthma?

Dr. Perlmutter explained that many of these disorders are related to the microbiome which, as I have explained previously, is the bacterial environment in the GI tract that either keeps us healthy or, when not cared for properly, makes us sick. The microbiome consists of a trillion bacterial cells (outnumbers our cells by ten times) living in a symbiotic relationship with us. We provide food for the bacteria when we eat, and the bacteria provide us with many different benefits. As an example, gut bacteria makes vitamins and other substances we use to perform necessary chemical reactions resulting in the production of a brain hormone; this maintains the health of the GI track lining or inhibits the growth of pathogenic bacteria in our intestines.

To be more specific, the good bacteria that live in our intestinal tract maintain an environment (microbiome) that most of the time does not allow the growth of bad/pathogenic bacteria which can harm us in many ways. A perfect example of this system going awry is when we take an antibiotic and end up with diarrhea. The antibiotic might have been prescribed for an upper respiratory infection (URI) which kills the harmful bacteria causing this problem; yet, it also kills the good bacteria in the microbiome. Many of the antibiotics used today are broad spectrum antibiotics. They are not targeted to kill only one type of bacteria; therefore, they wipe out any bacteria in their path. As a result, the antibiotic taken for a common URI produces a side effect that becomes difficult to deal with in the short and long term. We need to start thinking about the use of antibiotics differently knowing that they affect the microbiome in many negative ways. We need to look at the microbiome as an integral part of our health and take care of it in a very intentional way. Dr. Perlmutter also highlighted how the microbiome develops at birth. I have read much about this and am intrigued with the understanding of how we come into the world plays a large and permanent role in our health and whether or not we develop certain diseases over our lifetime. The microbiome develops naturally when we are born vaginally and develops in a different way when a child is born via C-section. Passage through the vaginal/birth canal inoculates the child with specific bacteria that colonize (take up residence) in the GI tract for the child's life. When a child is born via C-section, he/she becomes colonized with different bacteria having the potential to increase the risk for certain illnesses. There is much research ongoing that looks at the association of specific bacteria in the microbiome and the development of autism, dementia, obesity and allergies. These studies have shown a correlation which has to make us think intentionally about the first minutes of life and how our decisions influence the health of our children.

Dr. Perlmutter emphasized that correlation does not mean causation. What this means is that a correlation between two things does not necessarily mean that one causes the other, but are related. He talked about the different bacteria in the GI tracts of children born in Africa versus Europe and the incidence of certain diseases. I have read several reports about the incidence of Attention Deficit Disorder (ADD) in the U.S. compared to other countries and have thought about the significant difference in the rates, wondering why this is so. Some of the reports point to a correlation between birth methods, which types of bacteria initially populate the GI tract and the incidence of disease. It makes me re-think and look at this situation differently and question if there is something we can do to decrease the incidence of ADD and other diseases.

Since I am passionate about the prevention of disease, I continue to ask what I can do to help myself, my patients, family and friends to avoid illnesses and disease. Again, I will use the example of taking an antibiotic for an URI. First, we must understand that a respiratory infection can be caused by bacteria as well as a virus; and, in many cases the cold/flu symptoms we develop are caused by a virus. Treatment, therefore, with an antibiotic which only kills **bacteria** will do us no good and only harm. Unfortunately, many folks come to the office with a predetermined notion they need an antibiotic when they have flu symptoms. A common scenario is when a person is diagnosed with a viral infection; and, the physician tells the patient they need to rest, take a mild over-the-counter pain relief medication as necessary and the infection will resolve in a few days. The individual becomes unhappy since they believe that an antibiotic is necessary and often insist on getting a prescription. When this occurs, the unnecessary use of the antibiotic can harm not only the individual but also the community. The harm is widespread since wiping out good bacteria from the GI tract allows for the growth of pathogenic/ harmful bacteria that will eventually require stronger antibiotics to eradicate. The correct treatment is not to use an antibiotic in the first place knowing that our immune system is marvelously able to deal with viral and many other infections. In this case we allow the immune system to resolve the infection and at the same time do no harm to the microbiome. This becomes a win-win situation all around. The individual gets well, the microbiome remains strong and the community at large is not harmed. This new way of thinking about health care and looking at specific situations from a different perspective is how we can solve the health care problems that plague so many people today.

In closing, the message becomes protect and prevent. Protect the microbiome and prevent complications from unnecessary use of medications. Feed your gut bacteria healthy food and the trillions of bacteria in your system will help you in so many ways to stay healthy!

- Dr. Sal

Health Requires Being Intentional

When it comes to getting and staying healthy, intentionality rules! Being intentional requires lots of forethought and focus. It requires planning and deliberation; and, then tweaking and refining the plan until you get it just right. Sounds like a lot of work, right? Well, yes it is. Is there anything better than good health? Yes, great health! That's the goal. Optimal health, great fitness and over the top functionality lets you not give in to aging. Let's be intentional in our efforts to stay well.

Picture a day in the life of a person who lives health intentionally. He/she wakes up at a certain time each day to start planning with health as the number one priority. He focuses on doing things that improve health, thereby enabling him to do all the things necessary plus other activities he wants to do in the next 24 hours. Meals are intentionally planned. A lot of thought goes into deciding what to eat starting with breakfast which might be a bowl of oatmeal with berries and cinnamon along with a cup of green tea or a large glass of water. A second choice may be a veggie stir fry with wheat toast. Sounds yummy!

On the other hand, when she gets up in the morning, she focuses on getting her exercise done. She arrives at the gym by 5:30 am, works out doing 30 minutes of strength training and aerobic exercise for another 30 minutes before going home to a healthy breakfast to be ready for the day. If she prefers not to have a gym membership, she does an exercise video at home and uses some hand weights, resistance bands or some other method of strength training.

Both individuals understand the importance of healthy nutrition and regular exercise. Both are intentionally focused on each part of life. They prioritize these two behaviors understanding they are the foundation for healthy living. Throughout the day they ask themselves if what they are doing/eating promotes or detracts from good health. They are keenly aware that the decisions they make each day affect present and future health; and, they are not willing to take chances on losing health.

Intentionality requires planning...planning meals, scheduling exercise in the calendar, knowing the time to get to bed rather than leaving it up to chance. These are the day-to-day plans; in addition, these folks also plan social time, vacations, quiet time to reflect and think. They do not forget to do their wellness checks to be sure there are no early warning signs of disease. They ask for advice from their health care providers on how to stay well and how to age fitfully. When they visit their physician or health care provider, they want to know their numbers: blood pressure, weight, body fat percent, blood test numbers for lipids and glucose to name a few. When asked "how many minutes per day do you exercise?" and "how many servings of vegetables per day do you eat?" they know the answers; even more importantly, they know the importance of the questions. They also know the 5-2-1-0+9 rule for their children and are intentional on following these recommendations: five servings of vegetables daily, no more than two hours of play screen time (computer/TV), one hour of exercise daily, zero sugary drinks and nine hours of sleep nightly. They know children need more sleep than most adults. They are intentionally making sure their children are growing up healthy and again, not leaving it to chance.

Someone recently said to me, "failing to plan means you are planning to fail" and I believe this, especially when it comes to health. When we fail to plan to stay well, we eventually become sick. We will then have to plan visits to the doctor/hospital, plan finances so we can pay these tremendous bills, plan for someone to help us since failing health makes us less functional, and in some cases, plan funerals when catastrophic health problems occur. Please intentionally remember that most of the health problems we hear about today are preventable including heart disease, strokes, diabetes and cancer. These are not age-related illnesses; and, even when genetics puts us at risk, we must understand that genes are not our destiny. With healthy living we can keep these bad genes turned off. We do not have to succumb to genetics or unhealthy behaviors. We can do something about this every day. We can choose to be well and choose not to be sick. We can choose a life of pleasure and not pills. With each decision we make, we come closer to better health or closer to disease and disability. When we are intentional, we are in control!

One of the things I do with my patients is develop an action plan for healthy living. We intentionally write out a nutrition program, exercise schedule and sleep routine. We talk about ways to relieve stress and ways to live life with passion, dedication and commitment. We develop a plan to control life rather than having life control us.

In closing, I hope that you too will develop your own intentional action plan for healthy living. Take control of your health and define your future. Have fun and live life to the fullest.

- Dr. Sal

Are Low Fat Diets Really Helpful?

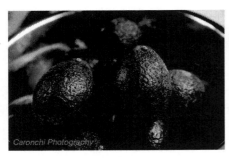

Caronchi Photography

With the low-fat craze, it seems we might be more at risk for getting less healthy; why is this occurring? What are many people eating in substitution for higher fat foods; and, does the low-fat eating have any negative consequences when it comes to overall health? What are fats used for anyway? There are many questions when it comes to the topic of fats in the diet, so let's understand the good and bad about fats starting with the classifications.

Fats are either saturated or unsaturated which relates to the relative health of this food category. Saturated fats are found in animal products, coconut and palm oil. Monounsaturated fats are found in olive oil, avocados, almonds, cashews and other nuts. Polyunsaturated fats occur in sunflower seeds, hemp, soybean, sesame and flax oil. In addition to these categories, we can classify fats as being inflammatory or not. We know that fats that come from animal products are more inflammatory and therefore less healthy. Good fats found in avocados and nuts are healthy for the brain, heart and other vital organs. Once we understand the categories, we can look at the functions of fats which include providing structural support for the cells, as an energy source and as a precursor for all hormones. Some fats such as the omega-3 fatty acids found in fish and fish oil decrease the risk of irregular heart rhythms and also decrease blood pressure. Fats make substances called prostaglandins which play a role in the body's inflammatory response to injury, allergies and infections. Fats are necessary for the function of the mitochondria, the powerhouses for energy production in all cells.

If we eat a very low-fat diet, deficiencies may occur; this is manifested as dry skin, brittle nails, decreased memory, an impaired immune response, decreased vision, mood swings, slow wound healing, heart disease and even depression. Treatment of fatty acid deficiency is preferentially through diet but sometimes supplements are necessary. Biotin, B12 and zinc are necessary supplements involved in the metabolism of fatty acids. That is why we need to be sure we are getting enough of these essential elements in the diet or as supplements.

Fatty acid deficiencies may also occur when we eat trans fats and when we eat too much sugar. Trans fats are synthetically produced fats which interfere with the production of natural fats and are directly linked to heart disease. Trans fats do not occur in nature; instead, they are produced by the food industry to help food stay fresh longer. You can think of them as a preservative. Trans fats increase the bad cholesterol (LDL), triglycerides and increase the stickiness of platelets which increases the risk of blood clots. They also decrease the level of good/HDL cholesterol. Trans fats may also decrease the stability of cell membranes allowing toxins to get into the cells. Most food product labels are now required to list the amount of trans fats. It is important to realize that any food product that contains hydrogenated or partially hydrogenated fats contains trans fats - avoid these also.

Sugar interferes with the enzymes that make fatty acids in the body; and, since we know that most Americans get too much sugar from what they eat and drink, we can understand how fat metabolism becomes a problem with the high sugar load from the standard American diet. Sugar (glucose) is necessary as an immediate source of energy yet excess sugar ends up being converted and stored as fat. Even more problematic is the fact that excess glucose in the body attaches to proteins and disrupts the normal function of these proteins. These sugar-protein complexes are called advanced glycation end

45

products (AGEs) and are associated with many diseases including dementia as well as premature aging.

The standard American diet is higher in inflammatory fats; therefore, tweaking the diet to get more Omega-3 anti-inflammatory fats is necessary. Eating wild fish a few times per week or taking a fish oil supplement is helpful. Also, eating a small amount of walnuts or other healthy nuts daily promotes good health. When we do not have the right balance of fatty acids, many different diseases may occur including heart disease, memory problems, psychiatric problems, gastrointestinal disorders, menopause symptoms, numbness/ tingling and even migraine headaches. As mentioned above and with other nutrition recommendations, we should be getting most of the fatty acids we need from the foods we eat. If we think we need to take fatty acid supplements such as fish oil, it is important to have a blood test first to measure the levels before making a decision.

When we look at what many people substitute for the fats that they decide not to eat, we see that they consume more carbohydrates and much of this is refined and processed. Eating too many types of bread, pasta, grains and other processed carbs will result in more sugar in the body along with more complications. The book, *Grain Brain*, by Dr. Perlmutter explains this mechanism well.

You may ask, when is it helpful to be on a low-fat diet and how should we change our nutritional intake to ensure we are eating the healthiest food? When a person has a history of a heart attack, stroke or other vascular disease, it is important to limit the bad fats, eat as much of the good fats as recommended; also, measure the types of lipids in the blood to make a difference in health for the short and long term. I have written articles about advanced lipid blood tests which measure the size and number of LDL cholesterol as well as the HDL, triglycerides and total cholesterol. With this additional information, the physician gets a better picture of the overall fat burden; therefore, the potential risk for cardiovascular disease as well as other metabolic diseases.

Once this information is known, a nutrition plan can be developed. The overall fat content should be about 10-20% of the total caloric intake with about 30-40% healthy protein and the remainder from non-refined, high quality carbs. The goal is to take in as much nutritionally dense foods as recommended. These are foods that are loaded with vitamins, minerals, antioxidants yet low in calories. For the best health, eat about six servings of vegetables daily, one or two fruits, non-processed carbohydrates with low glycemic load (so as not to quickly spike the insulin level in the blood) and healthy proteins, preferably from beans, nuts, lentils with limited amounts of red meat and processed lunch meats.

Also, remember to include daily exercise, stress management and sleep. The goal is to develop an action plan for healthy living with all these components which will result in optimal health and fitful aging. Especially during holiday celebrations, it is most important to remember these recommendations. Having an extra treat during the holiday season will not do much harm; while overdoing it in the long term will affect the quality and longevity of your life. Treat your body with kindness and love and it will return many gifts to you in each New Year and beyond.

- Dr. Sal

Making Sense of the Science

In preparing for a continuing medical education seminar one January, I had been reviewing the medical literature to better understand the health problems we deal with today in relation to traditional therapies and clinical outcomes. The focus of this review is what happens when we apply traditional medical treatments that often involve the use of prescription medications.

The health problems physicians and patients deal with today include elevated blood pressure, high cholesterol, heart disease, diabetes, obesity, dementia, musculoskeletal aches/pains and depression. If you watch television, you cannot miss the hundreds of commercials recommending medications to deal with these health problems. Do they really cure the problem, or do they simply treat the consequence of another underlying problem? As an example, high cholesterol is usually treated with medications such as a statin to bring down the numbers. What is the actual cause of the cholesterol elevation? In the United States this is most often (probably 90% of the time) related to a diet high in saturated fat. If the diet is not changed, taking the medication is like chasing your tail! This is similar to what happens when an asthmatic who smokes takes an inhaler to improve the shortness of breath. These treatments are directed at the consequence and not the cause.

Hypertension is another example. High blood pressure is often caused by hardening of the arteries or an excessive amount of adrenalin in the system. Anything that causes inflammation in the body affects the inner lining of the arteries (the endothelium) making the arteries less elastic and elevates the blood pressure. This creates strain on the heart which is now trying to pump blood against a higher pressure. Blood pressure medications are prescribed to lower the pressure; yet, many times the cause is not addressed nor corrected. When we look at the long-term benefits of treating high cholesterol with a statin or treating high blood pressure with an anti-hypertensive medication, do we find that these individuals actually live longer with less disease? Often the answer is no; this is usually because we have not alleviated the cause.

In looking at the clinical evidence, I have found hundreds of research reports which support the need to pay more attention to the cause and not the consequence. Many of these are listed in detail in Dr. Joel Fuhrman's book, *The End of Heart Disease*, and Dr. Michael Greger's book, *How Not to Die*. They discuss in great detail the fact that many of the health problems of today are man-made. Our lifestyle has created an epidemic of unhealthy individuals who spend the last years of their lives in sickness, not wellness. These lives are filled with medications, doctor visits, hospitalizations, disease, disability and early death. My apologies if this sounds morbid; this is the reality for many folks today. Because we often take health for granted, we do not cherish it and nourish it properly - then health fails! Trying to regain good health is much harder than keeping it in the first place.

The science also shows us that many traditional therapies (medications) often create as many problems as they solve. Again, let's take the statin medications as an example. They help lower cholesterol levels while increasing the risk for diabetes and in women some studies have reported an increased risk of breast cancer. There is also a concern they may increase the risk of age-related cognitive decline. For primary prevention (treating high cholesterol in a person who does not yet have heart disease), the studies do not show that a person actually lives longer as a result of this treatment. Are we simply exposing ourselves to side effects with no significant positive results? Wouldn't it be more appropriate to lower the amount of saturated fat in the diet to see how this influences the cholesterol level? I can tell you with certainty – this works! In my clinic, I have about 250 people involved in the **CHIP** program (the Complete Health Improvement Program) a nutrition program emphasizing eating lots of vegetables and other natural foods, while eliminating the foods that elevate the blood cholesterol in the first place. In just nine weeks, many of these folks have significantly lowered their lipid levels, without medication! I am referring to lowering the total cholesterol levels by 70, 80 and even 100 points! In reviewing the literature, I have not yet found any head-to-head research studies comparing nutrition to medications; yet, I can report the real benefits seen with patients in this program. The same goes for hundreds of other patients I see in my weight management clinic where I make similar nutrition recommendations.

A commentary was made about the research report in the *European Journal of Preventive Cardiology* in 2013 stating that "conventional (dietary) advice falls short in offering significant long-term protection against disease." We need to understand the science behind medical recommendations and give thought to all available traditional and alternative therapies. It is important to compare the benefits and know the risks/consequences so we (the patient and physician as a team) can make the best decisions to influence present and future health. Science (clinical evidence) should highlight the best approach in dealing with a health problem and not just masking the problem. Heart burn is another perfect example. Many people suffer from this because of what they eat. Taking a pill of any color (purple or otherwise) does not treat the problem. It just places a Band-Aid on the wound. Science shows long term use of acid lowering medications can have detrimental effects on the bones and other areas of the body. If acid reflux is not treated properly, the individual is at increased risk for esophageal cancer. Unfortunately, the TV commercials minimize the health implications of chronic heartburn/reflux. This is not a benign problem and should be treated by eliminating the cause.

The purpose of this writing is to share the messages from the scientific world which support the recommendations for lifestyle management in the treatment and prevention of most of the chronic illnesses and even many of the common cancers. There is much anecdotal evidence to support lifestyle as the most important way to stay healthy. I see this every day in my clinic. When people do the right things in relation to what they eat and how often they exercise, they stay well - better than most with less disease and fewer risk factors for chronic illness!

In summary, the science and the anecdotal evidence (what we see happening to people depending on how they live) makes sense – eat nutritious foods daily, stay active every day, manage stress, get good sleep, laugh and have fun daily. Do not take life too seriously - don't sweat the small stuff – life is too short! Enjoy each day and share your blessings with others.

- Dr. Sal

Whole Grains and the Gastrointestinal Health

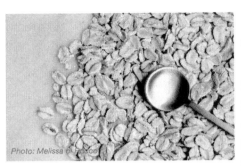

Photo: Melissa di Redfoot

The gastrointestinal (GI) tract is probably the most important interface the body has with the outside world. Certainly, the skin represents a large interface; since it is waterproof, it does not have the same important function as the GI tract which allows substances to cross into the blood stream. Another way to think about it: the lining of the GI tract decides what comes into the body via the blood stream and what does not. The cells that line the GI tract perform an amazing number of functions as they are exposed to a myriad of food particles, chemicals, toxins, bacteria and viruses. These specialized cells decide which substances traverse from the GI lumen into the blood stream and which need to be passed downstream into the large intestine on its way out of the body. The process by which the GI tract moves the contents downstream is called peristalsis; this process is aided by the fiber we eat and the fluids we drink.

Fiber comes in many different forms. Some are soluble and thereby absorbed, while some are insoluble and simply help the body form stool which rids it of waste products. Fiber is found mainly in vegetables, beans and grains. There is no fiber in meat products. Regular bowel movements (preferably daily) are important In order to have a healthy GI tract; this can occur when we eat lots of fiber and drink lots of water. This is one of the reasons an optimal diet should include several servings of raw and cooked vegetables daily, maybe a cup of beans and certainly whole grain breads or pasta.

When deciding on a bread product, confusion can set in since there are so many products to choose from; some are labeled whole wheat and others as whole grain. What is the difference? All grains start as whole grains which contain bran (the outer skin of the kernel), germ which has the potential to sprout into a new plant, and endosperm, the food supply for the germ. Whole grains are healthier because they contain all three parts.

Refining any grain product removes the bran and the germ leaving only the endosperm which then has only 75% of the original protein and has lost a significant amount of nutrients. If the reader is interested in learning what nutrients are lost in the processing of whole grains, I found a great graph on the website wholegrainscouncil.org.

When choosing a bread or pasta product, it is healthiest to choose a whole or intact grain. There are many to choose from including quinoa, barley, rye, buckwheat, brown rice, wild rice, amaranth and millet.

Quinoa is called a whole grain even though it is actually a seed which is high in protein. Barley is a whole grain which helps lower cholesterol. It is great in soups and can be mixed with rice and beans. Rye is often chosen by individuals with a gluten intolerance or sensitivity. It makes a great bread product. Brown rice is another whole grain which recently has fallen into disfavor since there is a concern about arsenic contamination. Wild rice is actually a grass seed and probably a better alternative to brown rice. Amaranth is high in protein and gluten free; therefore able to be eaten by those with celiac disease or gluten sensitivity. Millet is another gluten-free grain.

The key in the decision process is to choose a whole/intact grain in order to get the full benefit, eat enough soluble and insoluble fiber daily to help with absorption of nutrients; and, for the formation of normal, healthy bowel movements. The goal is to get about 40-50 grams of fiber per day, read the labels and keep track of your intake. If having a bowel movement is a problem, speak with your physician or health care provider about this. In addition to adding more fiber, you may need to take supplemental magnesium, add more water to your diet or get more exercise. Remember that bowel movements are the body's way of getting rid of waste products, toxins and other things that can make you sick.

When the colon is exposed to toxins for a prolonged time, it probably increases the risk for colon diseases and cancer. Also, when it comes to colon health, do not ignore the need to have a screening colonoscopy. Since colon cancers start as small polyps, which usually do not cause any symptoms, it is important to screen for early signs of colon cancer or colitis. Colonoscopies save lives! This is part of an optimal health approach which keeps the entire GI tract healthy. Please talk with your health care provider if you are older than 50 and have not yet had a colonoscopy.

The other disease which affects the GI tract commonly is heartburn, also known as reflux or GERD - gastroesophageal reflux disease. Actually, this should be more accurately described as a lifestyle induced health disorder rather than a disease. In most cases it is due to eating too much of the wrong foods that cause the GI distress. Unfortunately, commercials for the purple pill make it sound like you can eat anything you want; then, if heartburn occurs, simply take this acid-lowering pill to resolve the symptoms. It is important to understand that lowering the acid level in the stomach can result in bone loss, more susceptibility to infection, decreased absorption of certain essential vitamins and other health problems. The cure is not to eat foods that cause the heartburn in the first place! Reflux of acid into the esophagus increases the risk for esophageal cancer. Lifestyle behavior change is the answer and the solution which allows the entire GI tract to remain healthy.

- Dr. Sal

Diabetes and Persistent Organic Pollutants (POPS)

O ver the last 15-20 years we have seen an epidemic rise in the incidence of diabetes as well as obesity; and, we know the two are related to the point where now the term diabesity is often used in clinical literature. Previously, it was thought that being overweight was due primarily to excess consumption of calories and inactivity. Now we also know that the quality of food over the past several decades has dramatically diminished; therefore, could it be something in the food that has created this epidemic of diabesity?

Many researchers believe the other cause of this combined disorder has to do with contaminants in the food also known as persistent organic pollutants (POPS). These are chemicals in the environment, in the water we drink, the fish or meats we eat, in the air we breathe or from the multitude of plastics we come in contact with. Unfortunately, we live in a chemical-laden society and daily we are exposed to hundreds, if not thousands, of different chemicals, all of which can potentially cause harm especially in combination with other chemicals. We treat our lawns and shrubs with many different weed killers and fertilizers; we clean our homes with chlorine-based chemicals; we deodorize ourselves with underarm and body spray; we apply color to our hair and nails and use facial cleansers and makeup containing even more chemicals. The list goes on and on; and, the chemical companies tell us these are all safe to use.

Research experiments are done to test the safety yet a tremendously important point to understand is that they are done in isolation. This means that one chemical is tested alone to see if it is harmful and the reports usually come back stating they are not. What about the exposure to multiple chemicals? Many tests by researchers, not working for the chemical companies, have been done testing the safety of multiple chemicals in combination; and, to no one's surprise, the evidence points more to harm than safety.

One theory of aging has to do with progressive shortening of the ends (telomeres) of the DNA, as I have written about in News-Press articles. Anything that shortens the telomeres ages us quicker. Synthetic chemicals are known to damage the DNA; and, when this occurs, we seem to be more susceptible to cancer and other chronic illnesses.

Does persistent exposure to chemical pollutants harm us to the point where we become obese diabetics with cancer? The research makes me believe we must pay strict attention to this and try to lessen our exposures. We can do this by consciously avoiding as many chemicals as possible. One way this has been accomplished in the last decade, is to make plastic bottles and other containers that are BPA free. BPA is a chemical found in plastics that has been shown in some studies to have harmful health effects. If this subject seems to be controversial, ask who did the study. Was it supported by a company that makes plastics similar to the way many drug companies do safety studies? To truly evaluate the results of a research study, the design has to be unbiased. The researchers should have no vested interest in the results; should be searching for the facts. True scientific research is objective - the results should speak for themselves.

Another example of how society is attempting to lessen our chemical exposure is by producing meat products free of antibiotics, hormones and pesticides. Take a step back and ask how these chemicals get into our food supply in the first place and who made those decisions? Shouldn't we be aware from the start that doing something to our food supply is going to be harmful to the health of the population? Our main objective should be preventing illnesses; to cure disease. As we know, many of today's chronic illnesses and even cancers are stimulated by our behavior. What we do and how we live has such a tremendous impact on health and disease. We can either do things for ourselves (i.e., our food supply) to help us stay healthy; or, we can ignore the research, do the opposite and deal with the health consequences such as diabesity.

Research now is showing how antibiotics in our food supply affect the microbiome, the natural bacterial environment in our gastrointestinal tract that keeps us healthy. When we disrupt this by adding antibiotics to the food supply, we make it more difficult for our natural bacteria to survive and thus, keep us surviving. Also, the hormones that are administered to animals to make them grow fatter quickly are endocrine disrupters, meaning that they disrupt/affect in a negative way the normal hormone balance in humans. This is a very important point since we cannot live a healthy life without our hormones being in balance. As we get older, our natural hormones decline; and, this is one reason that many folks take supplemental hormones. Females, when necessary, should be supplemented with bio-identical estrogen, progesterone and any other hormones found to be deficient. For males, testosterone replacement (again with bio-identical and not synthetic hormones) makes them healthier and slows the aging process. When exposed to these synthetic endocrine disrupting hormones, the natural balance is thrown off, making it harder to remain healthy.

What can we do to avoid, as much as possible, these persistent organic pollutants, the endocrine disrupters and the multitude of other chemicals constantly bombarding us? The answer lies in our ability to live as clean as possible. On a daily basis, make a conscious effort to avoid the list of chemicals detailed above. If you eat meat, buy only grass-fed, antibiotic and hormone-free meat. Eat only organic fruits and vegetables to avoid the pesticides, buy them at the farmers markets where they cost less. Use household cleaners and body products which are less contaminated with chemicals. Limit foods that come in a box or a bag since most often they are filled with chemical preservatives, food coloring and other unnatural additives. Also, try to avoid GMOs (genetically modified) foods.

As I have recommended in many other articles, making good health your number-one priority every day helps you live a longer and better-quality life from a health perspective. There is nothing more important than your health - guard it, support it with healthy behaviors, and enjoy the rewards of taking the best care of your body and brain!

- Dr. Sal

Even a Plane Ride Can Teach You About Healthcare

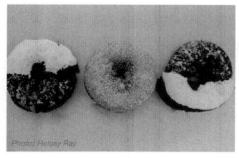

Photo: Helsey Ray

While flying to my home town in New York to celebrate a holiday with my family, I watched the documentary, *That Sugar Film,* which featured a young Australian man who decided to personally and intimately understand how sugar affects the human body. For 60 days he ate foods and drank beverages containing the average amount of sugar consumed by most adults in developed countries…40 teaspoons. The recommended limit for sugar consumption is six-nine teaspoons per day; therefore, it is clear that most adults intake considerably more sugar than necessary for energy production.

Before getting into the detrimental effects of too much sugar, the young man explains what sugar is used for (energy); and, what happens when you consume too much sugar (converted to fat and stored in the liver and around other vital organs). He starts eating typical foods rather than traditional junk foods. He avoids ice cream, candy and other foods high in sugar. Instead, he eats standard foods, even traditional foods served in school lunch programs. He has blood tests done at the start of his experiment and finds that they are all normal including liver blood tests; and, his physical examination with blood pressure, weight and abdominal waist measurements are all in the normal range.

Then, he starts eating what would be considered the standard American diet. To his surprise within just a few weeks, he starts to gain weight and belly fat, feels poorly and develops abnormalities in his blood tests including elevations in liver enzymes. When the liver enzymes elevate, this indicates there is damage to the cells in the liver. Medically, this is called non-alcoholic fatty liver disease (NAFLD) and the lay term is fatty liver. Often patients are made to believe that this is a benign condition; yet, in reality this is the precursor to liver cirrhosis and even liver cancer. NAFLD is a serious health problem.

Despite this, he continues with his experiment and continues to feel unwell. He becomes moody, noticing that his brain is not functioning normally; he continues to gain weight, gets sluggish and is now having difficulty tolerating his normal activity.

He notes that this is all occurring because he is having food and drink typically consumed on a daily basis by most adults. The rapid deterioration in his health amazes him as well as the physician and nutritionist he is working with. Together they calculate that he is eating the same number of calories he ate before the experiment started (2300 calories/day); but, he is now eating different foods and drinking different things that he had not previously. He notes before the experiment how he ate healthy fats such as avocados and nuts, proteins from fish or lean meats and limited sugary foods and drinks. His nutrition went from eating more natural foods to now eating mostly processed foods with the result being his health has declined rapidly and seriously.

Over this short period of time, he essentially develops what is known as metabolic syndrome, a combination of high cholesterol, blood sugar, blood pressure, weight gain in the abdominal area and also around the vital organs. This increases his risk for heart and blood vessel disease, diabetes, obesity and even cancer. In a short 60 days he goes from being a healthy young guy to a sick, debilitated person with significant health problems.

In addition to being curious about the health consequences, he also wants to understand how this is allowed. He questions the clinical research and the financial funding of research studies that in the past have come to the conclusion that sugar is really not a health problem.

60

He finds to his dismay that many of the research studies have been funded by corporations profiting from the sale of sugar, processed and other junk foods and drinks.

What this documentary reveals is what has happened to many Americans and others in developed countries over the past three to four decades. Since the 1950s, food has gone from being naturally grown to now being chemically produced. Profits have trumped health, and many have turned a blind eye to the damage this has produced, not only to the population but also to the planet. We no longer look at food as nutrition meant to keep us healthy. Instead, we now look for fast and convenient foods to quickly fill us up and disregard what is actually in the food and how it affects our health. The typical American now is over fed but malnourished. Obesity has become the norm; and, chronic illness such as diabetes, heart disease and cancer has replaced the infectious illnesses which caused most deaths and disabilities in the early part of the last century.

Even more importantly, this documentary revels that these problems are man-made! The health consequences of this young person's actions are brought on directly by what he does each time he sits down for another meal. He is ultimately killing himself with food!

At the end of the 60 days, he has his final blood tests and physical examination to fully understand what has happened. He made himself sick and tired by living the standard America lifestyle. Fortunately, he ends the experiment and goes back to eating healthy food again and in a few months his health returns to normal. This experience teaches us a lot. We must pay attention to what we feed ourselves and our children. We must pay attention to the importance of growing and eating healthy, nutritious food and not producing frankenfoods that destroy our health. We must not allow corporate profits to disregard the need for providing foods to the population which enhance longevity. Health is and should always be the number one priority; because, when we let it slip away, it is really hard to get back.

In closing, I recommend watching, *That Sugar Film*, to influence your decision in regards to what you eat and drink - I know I can do better! Each time I watch such a documentary, I learn more and get more motivated to cherish the health I have been given; and make sure I nurture it to live long enough to take more plane trips.

- Dr. Sal

Over 100 People Took The Pledge!

O ver 100 people took the pledge! On January 9, 2016, over 100 physicians, nurse practitioners, nurses, dietitians, hospital administrators, and others participated in the first annual Food is Medicine conference and took a pledge to talk honestly and openly with patients, family and friends about the ability of food to either create health or disease. This meeting was a milestone for our community. These wonderful people took four hours from their Saturday morning to hear how using food can save lives.

The program started at 7:30 a.m. with a healthy breakfast of quinoa, hummus, berries, fruits and vegetables. At 8 a.m., Dr. Brian Taschner, a cardiologist [from Fort Myers, FL], discussed many of the research reports linking food to the number one killer in the U.S., cardiovascular disease. He talked about the direct association of the standard American diet and the development of endothelial dysfunction and how inflammation within the walls of the arteries results in heart attacks, strokes, vascular disease in the legs and even Alzheimer's disease. He also detailed the many clinical reports proving the potential of healthy nutrition to treat, prevent and even reverse these chronic illnesses. He referenced, *The China Study*, by Dr. T. Colin Campbell, which documents the strong and direct relationship between chronic disease, cancer and food. Dr. Taschner gave examples of nutrition programs which enable people to live a better quality and longer life; he also talked about the Jumpstart program he is running. He provided solutions and took the pledge.

Next to present was Dr. Jose Colon, a specialist in sleep disorders and neurology for Lee Physician Group. He started with a great story to highlight the cause of many of the illnesses we deal with today. He helped the audience understand the importance of dealing with the cause of an illness and not simply trying to deal with the consequences of poor nutrition. His story and presentation allowed us to see the importance of breaking down walls and barriers, seeing a situation from another person's perspective and developing solutions to problems with this new found information. His message was, there is a better way; and, the way to better health is through better nutrition. He provided solutions and took the pledge.

After Dr. Colon finished his presentation, we took a ten-minute break for everyone to stretch, interact, drink some healthy water and get their minds reset for another two hours of learning. There was so much excitement in the room it was palpable. I have been to many conferences over my 22 years in medicine, rarely have I seen so much engagement and conversation, especially on a Saturday morning!

Around 10:15, Dr. Sebastian Klisiewicz took the microphone and started by showing the audience a picture of him and his son at the breakfast table having a healthy meal. He talked about the importance of teaching our children about healthy living and showed how he makes breakfast fun as his son eats his food with super hero action figures on the table. They talk about having a super hero breakfast together! Dr. Klisiewicz is a specialist in physical medicine and rehabilitation. He emphasized he is not a pain doctor; he treats pain with rehabilitation that involves diet and exercise. In reality he helps patients relieve pain by treating them with physical therapy, healthy nutrition, getting the toxins out of their bodies, weaning them off medications that often have more side effects than beneficial results, and by helping them emotionally through their illness. He treats the whole person and helps them understand the cause of their disability is frequently reversible by improving their lifestyle. Dr. Klisiewicz provided solutions and took the pledge.

After each of these presentations, the doctors took questions from the audience, and there were many. The people asked intelligent, probing and sometimes challenging questions; and, with each answer they were directed back to the science of nutrition. Each presenter was clear to make the audience understand that the context of their talk was not the physician's personal preference but rather a culmination of the objective scientific evidence supporting the relationship between food and health.

In combination, the three physician's presentations detailed hundreds of research reports making it absolutely clear that food causes chronic illnesses (cardiovascular disease, diabetes, obesity, Alzheimer's, musculoskeletal problems, etc.) and many of the common cancers. They also made it clear that healthy nutrition and an active lifestyle resulted in less disease and a longer life. They presented the facts and gave the audience solutions to the cause of illness.

At the end of each hour we had a drawing for Dr. Michael Greger's book, *How Not to Die*. Dr. Greger is a nationally renowned authority on healthy eating. As I told the audience, this book is full of objective, clinical research about the science of nutrition. Personally, I have no vested interest in this book but recommend it highly for anyone interested in learning more about food and health. Dr. Greger, like the three physicians who presented at the conference, emphasizes Food is Medicine and our medicine tastes a lot better than the pill medicines most Americans swallow each day.

Next to the microphone was Yours Truly. Public speaking is one of the best parts of my job - I love talking about health and helping people understand that getting older does not mean we have to grow old with disease. There are many ways we can age with vitality. From personal and professional experience, I know that healthy eating, exercise and a healthy lifestyle allows a person to age in a functional and fit way. With the microphone in hand, I reviewed my slide presentation which was intended to help the audience see the relationship between disease and lifestyle. It is clear to me that many of the illnesses people suffer with today are man-made. Health care providers often prescribe treatment that comes in the form of a pill. Many times this treatment does not address the cause of the illness;

and, in addition to some benefit, also brings many side effects or complications. Now the physician and the patient must deal with more than the original problem. The initial man-made health problem is given a treatment which creates another man-made problem we again have to treat.

The substance of my presentation was to focus on the cause of the illness. The research I presented proved that many of our health problems come from eating unhealthy food; it showed that when we prioritize health by eating mostly healthy, nutritious food, we live the life most people in this country yearn for. When I finished discussing the clinical research regarding health and nutrition, I talked with the audience about many of my patients (no names divulged) who have had remarkable success in treating, preventing and reversing disease via healthy nutrition. I detailed dozens of patient statistics showing how weight, BMI, body fat, blood pressure and blood test results improved as each person started eating healthy food. Sounds simple? Well, IT IS! I reviewed some of the results of the **CHIP** program (Complete Health Improvement Program), an instructor facilitated program, which teaches people how to shop for, cook and eat healthy food; and, how well participants in this program do in just nine weeks.

At the end we passed out lapel pins displaying an outline of an apple with the words, Food is Medicine. As a team, Drs. Taschner, Colon, Klisiewicz and I asked the audience to recite with us the pledge if they were to wear this pin and the pledge as follows:

> *"I pledge to wear this Food is Medicine pin to talk honestly and openly with patients, family and friends about the ability of food to either create health or disease; and, by engaging people in this conversation, I will be able to help them improve their lives while decreasing the risk of disease and disability."*

It was awesome to see and hear over 100 people stand and proudly recite this statement - one of the highlights of the event for me! I want to thank the physicians and all the others who worked hard preparing for this event. Many thanks to all who attended and will now help us champion our cause as we continue to make ourselves, our family, friends, patients and our community healthier by using *Food is Medicine.*

- Dr. Sal

Can Watching Movies Make You Healthier?

Recently I watched The Martian, a movie which was enjoyable and even educational since it depicted highly intelligent people continually solving problems. Matt Damon plays an astronaut stranded on Mars alone for over 500 sols - or Martian days. Almost from the minute he becomes stranded, problems develop which must be solved if he is going to survive. After he does some minor surgery on a puncture wound in his abdomen, he next has to figure out how he is going to feed himself for an unknown period of time. He knows he has only a finite amount of food rations and therefore has to figure out how to grow food. After this, he has to figure out how to make water; and the problems continue to pop up, so he has to continue to think logically and, even more so, scientifically.

This is where the education comes in as it relates to health. I wrote a News-Press article about the medical seminar Dr. Colon, Klisiewicz, Dr. Brian Taschner and I presented which focused on the scientific link between nutrition, health and disease. We emphasized throughout the four-hour seminar that we were presenting the scientific evidence and not our personal preferences. The Martian movie highlighted how science is able to solve problems, keep a man on Mars healthy and alive. Our seminar highlighted how men, women and children can use science to stay alive and healthy. The latter word, healthy, is the important point.

Many people in this country are alive but not healthy. Most people over 50 live with at least one chronic illness and take at least one medication daily. The norm as we grow older is more medication, more illness, more disability and less functionality. Wow - that's a lot to look forward to! We work all our lives only to end up sick and debilitated. This is not our destiny; we are not genetically programmed to get sick and die early. Science has shown that through healthy living we can live until 90 and even over 100 years. If you do not believe this statement, there are books and articles to read about people who live in Blue Zones® : Ikaria, Greece; Sardinia, Italy; Loma Linda, California; Okinawa, Japan; and Costa Rica. These people abide by the science of healthy living without even knowing it. They eat natural, unprocessed food, are active every day, socialize; and, have strong family and community support. They laugh and live very differently than many people in other parts of the world. Dan Buettner, an author of Blue Zone® books, has been studying the folks living in these beautiful areas of the world and has looked closely at the science surrounding their ability to live so long.

Another person who looks critically at the science of health is Dr. Michael Greger, a nationally known author and educator in the area of health, wellness and nutrition. If you have not looked at his website, www.nutritionfacts.org, I highly recommend it. This site is filled with unbiased, scientifically based information which explains the link between what we eat and how healthy we age. The focus is on the science and not his personal preferences on eating. He even states this in his new book, How Not To Die. He acknowledges when people ask him to describe what he eats, he answers by stating that another person should not follow his way of eating rather, follow a nutritional approach that has been shown scientifically to result in better health. The emphasis is on the science. When we think about it, science is so exciting, educational and rewarding. The Martian movie simply highlights how people can use science to solve problems. Dr. Greger reminds us of the same. In our presentations, Drs. Colon, Klisiewicz, Taschner and I did the same. So…you can see movies and learn about science and health!

In my role as the VP of Health & Wellness for the Lee Memorial Health System [at the time of this writing], I am passionate about spreading the message: there is a better and a healthier way to live. If we follow the science, we will have the knowledge to make the best decisions on a daily basis, improve the quality of our lives; and, as science shows, will improve our chances of living longer!

- Dr. Sal

Why Change Now?

Change is difficult - we all know that and have had to make decisions to change at certain times in life. Many of life's events require change and how we deal with this can impact us in small and large ways. When it comes to health and wellness, we make decisions daily which impact our present and future health; when we need to make a change because of failing health, it is still difficult.

This scenario is the most frustrating one for health care providers. Let me explain further with a few true stories using fictitious names. Bill was a middle-aged patient of mine who owned a very profitable company, which was going to be bought out by one of the largest companies in the world making Bill a very rich person. While Bill worked very hard at his job, he spent less effort on the diabetes he had for many years. Each time I saw Bill in my office, I would emphasize the need to focus on managing his diabetes, yet most of the time Bill did not heed my warnings. During one of his last visits, I advised Bill to pay close attention to managing diabetes, or pay the consequences! Bill's wife was in full agreement with my approach, but Bill did not heed my warnings. He refused to change believing that nothing bad would come of his non-compliance. Unfortunately, Bill was wrong. A short time after this visit, he developed chest pain, went to the emergency room, had a massive heart attack and died. His refusal to change had a major impact on his life and the lives of so many others who loved him.

Another patient who refused to change was Sam. Sam and his wife had the type of marriage that so many couples wish they had. These two people adored one another, and their love was obvious. Sam also had a chronic illness that was impacting his present life and I

71

told him many of the same things I told Bill. I would say, "Sam you are not listening to me. Your unwillingness to change lifestyle behaviors will sooner or later catch up with you and I do not want to see that happen. You have a lot to live for so why not make the necessary changes, so you can become and stay healthy?" Sam would answer by saying, in effect, that change was hard. What he did not realize was that his current lifestyle would force him to change at one time or another. Sickness forces you to change in ways that are out of your control. Sickness does not care that you have a multi-million dollar company to run or if you have a wife and family that adore you. Sickness makes everything change. Sam ended up having a heart attack in the garage when he and his wife were cleaning, leaving his beautiful wife devastated. She believed he was too selfish to change and now she also was paying the price.

One final true story not quite as sad is that of Cynthia who thought she was healthy until she had a stroke. Cynthia was another patient with less than optimal compliance with her health care. She was too busy to do the simple things she needed to do to stay well. She got what she describes as her wakeup call when she acutely suffered a stroke leaving her weakness in her arm and leg as well as difficulty with her memory. Her stroke, fortunately, was not fatal but the loss of physical and mental function was permanent, as was the change this illness had on her life. She now feels she is a burden to her family and is dealing with the guilt for not taking better care of herself.

This is the reason I am so passionate about preventive health care. Every day I see patients like Bill, Sam and Cynthia and give the same recommendations…you can take control and change now in order to live a healthier life; or, you can change later on, when a chronic Illness or cancer forces you to change. Once this occurs, it is much harder to regain good health. The answer to the question, Why change now?, becomes apparent. When it comes to health, change is often the best option. Many people living in this wonderful country live a very unhealthy lifestyle. When sickness occurs, these same people are willing to make radical changes. They are willing to undergo open heart surgery, take chemotherapy, use multiple medications daily and even change what they eat and how they exercise. It is obvious that most of us have the capacity to change.

The take-home message from this article is clear - do not wait to change! Make the necessary changes in relation to health and wellness starting today; stay on the path of optimal health. Let's do this together so we can all look forward to a bright future filled with good health and vitality!

- Dr. Sal

So...What's The Cause, Doc?

Over the years I have had many patients diagnosed with high blood pressure, high cholesterol, Alzheimer's, reflux, chronic low-back pain and many other ailments. Occasionally the patient will ask, "so... what's the cause?" With this question, the individual has gotten to the heart of the matter.

Current medical care usually proceeds as follows: a person is diagnosed with high blood pressure or another disorder and is most often treated with a medication. The time lapse between diagnosis and the written prescription being handed to the person is short; and, the amount of time spent trying to identify the cause of the high blood pressure or other medical problem is limited. This appears to be one of the major realities of medical care today. We often do not look hard enough to identify the cause; then, when found, not enough is done to remove the cause. We simply treat the symptom.

This process creates several more problems the health care provider and patient must deal with. To begin with, the reason for the health problem, the high blood pressure, is not identified. While the medication prescribed provides some relief from the high blood pressure, it also has side effects. Essentially, there are no medications without side effects. Even an aspirin has side effects; therefore, the automatic prescription brings benefits as well as potential complications. When complications arise, often another prescription is written to deal with that. The cycle continues until we identify the cause and remove it.

Let's take cholesterol as another example. An individual is diagnosed with high cholesterol. The usual treatment is a prescription for a cholesterol-lowering medication and some quick advice about

74

eating better. The patient walks out of the office, in many cases, with less than a clear understanding of what to do regarding nutrition. Even more importantly, he/she does not understand the importance of the need to change lifestyle behaviors in order to truly treat the high cholesterol.

Gastrointestinal reflux is another great example. I loathe the commercial for the purple pill. The heavy-set actor eats all the wrong foods and then recommends to the audience to take this purple pull to relieve the heartburn symptoms. Maybe he should stop eating the foods that cause the symptoms! Even more irresponsible is the fact that this commercial makes light of GI reflux, a potentially life threatening condition. Chronic heartburn means stomach acid is continually moving up into the esophagus where it is not supposed to be. This exposes the lining of the esophagus, increasing the risk of bleeding and cancer formation. When acid refluxes up into the back of the throat, it can be inhaled into the lungs causing wheezing as well as other pulmonary complications. Often when this occurs, the person is prescribed an inhaler medication to deal with the wheezing. Once again, more medication is prescribed to treat the complications of an unhealthy lifestyle. Why not just stop eating the foods which cause the reflux so the GI problem, as well as the lung problems, are solved?

The above examples make it apparent that we must identify the cause of a health problem in order to truly treat it. Treat the cause, not just the symptom. For most health problems, the common denominator is inflammation. In past News-Press articles I have emphasized this and also in my public presentations. From heart disease, Alzheimer's and arthritis, inflammation is the problem. If we look at cardiovascular disease, we know that inflammation of the inner lining of the arteries starts the process of plaque formation which eventually leads to obstruction of blood flow. Over time, the reduction in blood flow decreases the function of the organ it supplies; and, if a piece of this plaque ruptures, blocking all blood flow causing a heart attack, stroke or another serious circulatory emergency.

Inflammation in the brain is known to be part of the mechanism of dementia and other neurodegenerative diseases. The same is true for arthritis and many other musculoskeletal disorders. Studies have shown that people taking anti-inflammatory medications can have a lower incidence of these inflammatory conditions including a decreased risk of colon polyps. The explanation for this appears to be that polyps arise as a result of inflammation in the colon; and, reducing the inflammation decreases the risk and incidence of polyps.

How should we proceed when a health problem is diagnosed? We investigate all potential causes; and, once we are confident that we have found the answer, we do what is necessary to remove the cause. If a high-salt diet and lack of exercise is causing the high blood pressure, then we eliminate salt from the diet, get the person on an exercise program, help him/her lose weight if this is part of the problem and monitor the blood pressure. In some cases, even with these lifestyle changes, medication is still necessary; yet, as long as we are confident that we have dealt with the cause of the problem, we can then use blood pressure lowering medications more appropriately. The same goes for high cholesterol. In the CHIP (Complete Health Improvement Program) that we run for Lee Memorial Health System employees, many participants lower their cholesterol and get off medications simply by changing what they eat, how they exercise and by lowering their weight. I am not suggesting that this is simple to do. It takes work, but it is worth it!

There is nothing more important than maintaining good health. When health fails, all else in life fails. Optimal health should always be the number one priority; and, we should be intentional about what we eat, how we exercise and how we live, to safeguard our health. It is important to ask yourself: what am I doing that might be causing the symptom (high blood pressure, high cholesterol, or others)? What can I do to rectify this problem? Do I really need to take a medication and is this going to create more complications that I might have to deal with? Do I really understand the cause of my health problems and am

I willing to make the necessary lifestyle changes in order to live a healthier and longer life? These are all very important questions to think about, discuss with your physician or health care provider and answer with certainty.

In the past I have suggested that you watch the You Tube video, Make Health Last. This video will remind you of how many people in America spend the last ten years of their life - in sickness, not in wellness. It reminds us that it is important to grow older with vitality and not to grow old with disease since the latter shortens our lives and most definitely decreases the quality of the last years. After you have watched this video, work with your physician or health care provider to develop an action plan for healthy living. Focus on this action plan daily; it will enable you to do all the things you enjoy in life!

- Dr. Sal

Stroke – Another Cardiovascular Disease Equivalent

Recently there was a wonderful event, The Stroke Ability Fair, which highlighted services available in Lee County, Florida. It was geared toward helping people with a stroke to be more functional and focused on the ability of a person after a stroke. In this article, I will discuss stroke as a cardiovascular equivalent; a person who has suffered a stroke has the same risk for a heart attack or other circulatory disorders.

When someone has suffered a heart attack, stroke, a blood clot in the leg or lung, they have vascular disease known as endothelial dysfunction. In all these conditions, the inner lining of the arteries (the endothelium) and veins are inflamed; and, if the inflammation is not reversed and resolved as soon as it begins, the arteries become clogged with plaque and blood flow to all the cells in the body is diminished. When blood flow is decreased, there is a limitation of oxygen and nutrients getting to the vital organs. The organs (heart, kidneys and brain) become dysfunctional and the person as a whole ages more rapidly.

One of the most important things to remember about a stroke is that this is an emergency. When symptoms of a stroke develop, the individual must call 911 and get to the emergency room ASAP! Remember the terminology, stroke attack similar to a heart attack. When a person has chest pain, he/she calls 911 and is taken to the emergency room for specialized medication and treatment to stop the damage from progressing. The same thought process must be maintained with someone who is having a stroke.

The signs and symptoms of a stroke are sudden and can include weakness in an arm or leg, slurred speech, difficulty swallowing,

78

drooping of one side of the face or one corner of the mouth, dizziness or problems walking, slow word finding and vision problems. Realize that not all these symptoms occur simultaneously; any combination of these may represent a stroke. When this occurs, the person needs to get to the emergency room immediately.

Transport to the emergency room must be done via ambulance. In over 20 years of practicing internal medicine, I have knowledge of two patients dying in the car when they insisted that a family member drive them to the emergency room. This is a major mistake that turned into a fatal mistake. While in the ambulance, the emergency medical professionals can start treatment and talk with the ER physician to let him/her know what is happening. In this situation treatment starts immediately and the stroke victim is in good hands. In contrast, if the person having a stroke insists on someone driving them to the ER and the situation gets worse, there is nothing that can be done. Please heed these warnings.

Strokes can occur for several different reasons. One is when a blood clot travels to the brain and lodges in a small artery blocking the blood flow to a particular part of the brain. This clot often comes from a blood clot which has formed in the heart; or, it comes from arterial plaque which breaks off and travels to the brain. These are called embolic strokes. They basically represent vascular or heart disease which then affects the circulation in the brain. Some people with atrial fibrillation develop cardio-embolic strokes. This is because the top part of the heart (the atria) fibrillates rather than pumping normally. The blood in the heart can clot and then a piece of this clot can travel into the brain.

When the carotid arteries (the large arteries which supply the brain) become inflamed, endothelial dysfunction occurs. If this persists, plaque builds up along the wall of the artery; if this plaque ruptures, a piece of this plaque travels to the brain and occludes (blocks) one of the small arteries. In both situations, it is the occlusion that creates the problem.

The other type of stroke is called a hemorrhagic stroke; this occurs when a small blood vessel in the brain ruptures allowing blood to leak into the brain tissue. Hemorrhagic strokes occur commonly in people with uncontrolled hypertension (high blood pressure) and in others who have a malformation of an artery or an aneurysm which is an abnormal swelling of part of the artery/vein. The brain is contained in the skull and as such has a finite amount of room. When blood leaks into the brain, it puts pressure on the brain and causes it to malfunction. Symptoms of either an embolic or a hemorrhagic stroke are similar; although, if the bleeding continues into the brain, the symptoms of a hemorrhagic stroke can be more severe. As pressure builds up in the brain cavity, the brain can be pushed downward affecting the breathing centers of the brain. In this situation, the stroke can be fatal. Once again, it is vitally important for the person to get to the ER via ambulance, so the physician can make the correct diagnosis.

Although some of the symptoms are similar, the treatment is different. The embolic stroke is usually treated with medications to get rid of the clot. In the case of a hemorrhagic stroke, the treatment has to deal with the bleeding and pressure on the brain.

While in the hospital, the initial treatment is described above; once the emergency treatment stops progression of this disease, the next step is to assess the overall damage and start rehabilitation. A person suffering a stroke might be left with impaired speech or significant weakness in an arm or a leg, making walking difficult. Others might have persistent double vision or chronic dizziness. Some symptoms are even more severe while for some, all symptoms resolve within a short period of time. Once the damage is apparent, a plan for rehabilitation can be designed. This can involve a speech therapist, a traditional physical therapist, or may require a psychologist since some people develop depression after a stroke. This might occur in a person with persistent physical problems after a stroke that previously was

80

fully functional. It is often hard to cope with a disability; and, this might create psychological distress requiring counseling and other types of emotional support.

      With time, many people learn to become functional again. It is important to realize that a person after a stroke has many abilities. Some people regain full functionality both physically and mentally. Support from health professionals, family and friends will be most important to encourage the person so he/she understands this. With help and hard work many patients get back to normal living. It is most helpful to be positive; however, in the situation where full functionality is not attained, it is helpful for the stroke victim to know that services are available to make life easier.

- Dr. Sal

Understanding the Importance of Detoxification

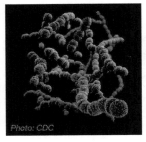
Photo: CDC

Have you ever thought about how the body gets rid of toxins? When you look around, the environment we live in is filled with toxins — from the air we breathe to the water we drink. Toxins come to us in the form of food which is often contaminated with hormones, antibiotics, pesticides as well as fecal bacteria and viruses in red meat and chicken, cancer causing nitrosamines in lunch meats and pesticides/herbicides on fruits and vegetables. We are also exposed to many thousands of chemicals in the myriad of processed foods that come in a box or a bag. When we are outside in the sun (a little sun is necessary for Vitamin D production), radiation is another toxin that we know affects the DNA and increases the risk for cancer. Next, there are a slew of chemicals which we are exposed to in the plastic bottles we drink from, the clothes we wear, the dry cleaning solutions used to clean our suits and dresses. Gasoline and the exhaust fumes when inhaled are other sources of toxins. Let's not forget tobacco smoke and the chemicals we clean our homes with or the weed killers we put on our lawns! The list goes on and on. In reality we are exposed to hundreds if not thousands of toxins on a regular basis and all need to be acted upon by our defense mechanisms if we are to stay healthy.

Detoxification occurs in many areas of the body including the liver, lungs and the colon. Many toxins arrive within us from the foods we eat and liquids we drink. The colon has the job of deciding which substances will enter the body and which will be eliminated in the stool or urine. We know that the bacteria within the colon help with the detoxification process; and, these healthy bacteria also

82

produce vitamins and other nutrients that keep the lining of the GI tract healthy. We can consider the GI tract the first line of defense. In actuality, the large majority of the immune cells are within the GI tract. This is one reason it is so important to keep the GI tract and the microbiome healthy. The microbiome is the environment within which the healthy bacteria of the gut live. We need to feed these bacteria with healthy food, so they continue to keep us (the host) healthy. Maintaining normal, frequent bowel movements (at least one per day) is essential to remove toxins from the colon.

The next level of detoxification occurs in the stomach and small intestine. Hydrochloric acid (HCL) made in the upper GI tract helps kill bacteria and other organisms that do us harm. When we take the purple pill to lower the acid production and stop heartburn, we decrease the ability of the GI tract to remove toxins and also negatively affect the health of our skeletal system.

Liver detoxification represents another level and consists of two phases. In phase one the toxins are acted upon by liver enzymes with the goal of making the toxins less harmful. In phase two these intermediate substances are further metabolized into water soluble forms that are then eliminated in the urine or stool. The production of all the enzymes used in these detoxification chemical reactions require vitamins, proteins, carbohydrates and minerals which must be supplied from the foods we eat and liquids we drink. Without proper nutrition, the body is unable to make the necessary enzymes for phase one and two liver detoxification reactions.

The metabolism of pharmaceutical medications is a good example of the need for proper liver detoxification defenses. All medications, even over-the-counter drugs, need to be metabolized, utilized and excreted. When the liver has to deal with metabolizing many drugs each day, it can become overwhelmed leading to less than adequate detoxification. The average American adult takes at least one prescription medication and many folks take up to five or more a day.

In this situation, the therapeutic levels of prescription drugs can be changed thereby altering the effect of the medication.

Many of these chemical reactions produce reactive oxygen species which we can think of as a substance capable of rusting cells from within (aka oxidation). When a person does not eat nutritious food and has a deficiency of antioxidants, these reactive oxygen species create havoc within cells, disrupting the ability to detoxify and even decreasing the cells ability to create energy for its own function. Free radical formation is also known to advance the aging process; and, as I have discussed in many of my previous articles, they also cause endothelial dysfunction making blood flow through the arteries more difficult.

In addition to eating nutritious foods, we can use supplements to support the detoxification pathways including B-complex vitamins, vitamins C and E, as well as amino acids which are necessary to make the detox enzymes. Healthy nutrition which helps in these reactions include whole grains, Brewer's yeast, fruits, vegetables, sprouted seeds, beans and other sources of protein. Trace minerals such as magnesium, zinc and others are also essential.

When we look at pharmaceutical medications as a toxin, we must realize that prescription drugs are primarily helpful; yet, they do place a burden on the detoxification system and all medications have side effects. It is sad but unfortunately true that properly prescribed medications represent the fourth leading cause of death in the U.S. accounting for about 100,000 deaths annually. I emphasize the word properly meaning that these medications are clinically necessary and appropriately prescribed, but have side effects and unintentional consequences. Many of these folks are hospitalized and the estimated cost is over $1 billion.

Now that we know the expansive but not complete list of toxins that affect us daily, what can we do about it? First, we need to live as clean as possible. This means trying to avoid or limit many of the toxins listed above as much as possible. Start with eating real food that has not been contaminated and the same with drinking water. Look critically at everything you come in contact with to see if there are ways to eliminate toxins from your environment. Next, support the detoxification pathways and the immune system with nutritional supplements as prescribed by a naturopathic, holistic or integrative medicine physician. Learn also how to support the microbiome. This means feeding the healthy bacteria in your GI tract and not feeding the pathogenic (disease causing) bacteria. One way to help the microbiome is to take antibiotics only when 100% necessary so as not to kill off the healthy bacteria which do so much to keep us well. After a course of completely necessary antibiotics, it is important to repopulate the GI tract with healthy bacteria by taking probiotics and pre-biotics (food for the bacteria). Consultation with a nutritionist would be helpful in this regard.

In preparing for this article, I read many research reports on the benefit of cruciferous vegetables in the detoxification process. These include broccoli, cauliflower, Brussels sprouts, cabbage and bok choy. These wonderfully healthy vegetables contain healthful chemicals which support the detoxification pathways and have been shown to decrease the risk of many cancers. Other healthful chemicals are found in green tea (ECGC), fruits (flavonoids) and in the Indian spice, turmeric (curcumin).

In summary, you can support the detoxification system by decreasing the toxic load, increasing the elimination of toxins in the urine and stool, supplying the body with healthy macro and micronutrients, increasing the efficiency of the liver function (limit alcohol, Tylenol and other medications or drugs which negatively affect the liver), supporting the gut bacteria (the microbiome) and making sure not to develop leaky gut syndrome by keeping the lining of the GI tract healthy.

It is amazing to understand the magnitude of the toxic burden we have to deal with each day; yet, it is even more amazing to know that our body is capable of keeping us well despite this daily barrage.

The body is truly amazing and, as long as you support it with a healthy lifestyle, it is able to afford you many decades of good health.

- Dr. Sal

Feed the Good Bacteria

There are many books and articles written recently about the microbiome, the internal environment in the gastrointestinal tract where millions of bacteria live in a symbiotic relationship with all human beings. From the many years of studying this, research has shown these bacteria are not just taking a free ride. They actually contribute to the health of the host (us) when they are injured, as when we take antibiotics, we become less healthy. Where do these bacteria come from and how do they get inside of us? They come from the environment and are inside of us starting at birth; and, how we are born affects which bacteria initially colonize our GI tract. When the bacteria is analyzed in the GI tract of a child born normally (vaginally), this child has different bacteria as compared to a child born via C-section. We have been designed over thousands of years for a natural vaginal birth. For various reasons, many children born in the last 50 years have been born via C-section, exposing the child to skin bacteria as compared to the child born vaginally who is exposed to birth-canal bacteria. Research has shown differences in the health of children born via these two approaches which can last for many years, if not the life of the individual.

After the child is born, it is also known that the method of feeding also affects which bacteria take up residence in the GI tract. Breast feeding versus bottle feeding affects the microbiome. Bacteria on the skin of the mother get into the child and populate the child's GI tract. Beyond this, it is known that breast milk contributes to better overall health for the child, since breast milk provides antibodies and other nutrients the child needs to start life in a healthy way. Breast feeding encourages a close bonding opportunity for the mother and child; therefore, there are a number of reasons to encourage breast feeding.

As the infant becomes a young child, what he/she consumes in addition to food affects the microbiome. In the early years of life a typical child in the U.S. receives many doses of antibiotics. It is known that antibiotics kill bacteria; when taken orally, antibiotics do not discriminate between the good and the bad bacteria within us. They kill all bacteria they come in contact with, meaning that they also kill the healthy bacteria within the microbiome. Since the bacteria within the microbiome contribute to our health, killing them off with antibiotics meant to treat a respiratory, urinary or other infection affects the recipient in a negative way. Essentially, the antibiotic helps for one problem --the acute infection, while it hurts in another way by negatively impacting the microbiome.

Let's review the beneficial effects of the GI flora --the bacteria living in the microbiome. The normal/healthy bacteria within the GI tract suppress the growth of abnormal/pathogenic/disease-causing bacteria. The normal bacteria also stimulate the immune system, reduce inflammation which strengthens the lining of the GI tract, help rid us of toxins and produce vitamins that we use to improve our own health. These are extremely vital functions which contribute to the health of the host; again, these internal bacteria live with us in a symbiotic relationship.

By watching television, one comes to understand the myriad of diseases and disorders which affect the GI tract. In addition to GERD, people often are afflicted by irritable bowel syndrome (IBS), different types of colitis such as Crohn's disease and ulcerative colitis, diverticulosis and diverticulitis, chronic constipation, infectious diarrhea, to name a few. These TV commercials recommend treatments which are often medications used to treat the symptom, not the cause. The commercial for the purple pill to treat heartburn only treats the symptom but does not highlight the reason for the heartburn which is what we eat and drink. By not eating and drinking things that give us the heartburn in the first place, we can avoid the GERD and avoid the side effects of the purple pill. This is common sense!

Many of the other diseases and GI disorders mentioned above would have a similar outcome. Our focus should be more on what we put in, and don't put in, our GI tracts through our mouths. Gluten sensitivity is another example. Many people are sensitive to protein in wheat and other grains causing GI problems such as abdominal pain, loose bowel movements, gas and bloating; yet, even more problematic is the weakness this causes in the lining of the GI tract which can lead to the leaky-gut syndrome. When the GI tract becomes leaky, toxins, bacteria and other harmful substances can cross from the lumen of the GI tract into the blood stream, causing a number of problems including allergies, inflammatory joint problems, asthma and more.

What should we supply the microbiome with in order for the bacteria to remain healthy? First, what we should **not** do is take antibiotics unnecessarily. Antibiotics are necessary when we have a **bacterial** infection; they do nothing for viral infections. When a person has the flu or another viral infection (many upper respiratory infections are viral), he/she should not take an antibiotic. This harms the bacteria within the GI tract that we need to stay healthy. When diagnosed with a bacterial infection and when antibiotics are necessary, after the course is completed, it is helpful to take a probiotic to help repopulate the GI tract with healthy bacteria. Since there are many probiotics on the market, it is best to look for one with at least 50 billion CFUs (colony forming units) containing lactobacilli and bifidobacterium. Most beneficial probiotics contain at least five to seven different strains of bacteria and are stomach coated in order for the live bacteria to get into the colon. The stomach coating inhibits stomach acid from killing the probiotics. It is important to read carefully the wording from the manufacturer which guarantees that the product was tested; and, that it contains the number of live bacteria stated on the label.

In addition to probiotics, it is helpful to supply **prebiotics** (food for the bacteria) such as oats, garlic, onions, banana, artichoke, leeks and asparagus. These are healthy foods which can be eaten any time of the day. Rolled oats in the morning with a cup of berries is a great way to start the day and keep the brain healthy. A good lunch might be a spinach salad with artichokes, garlic, onions, asparagus along with some avocado, walnuts and freshly ground flax seed for healthy fats. Meals such as these feed the good bacteria in the GI tract and in turn the bacteria feed you with vitamins and other chemicals needed to stay healthy.

There are many exciting books to read and learn more about the microbiome such as *Brain Maker*, by Dr. David Perlmutter; and, *The Microbiome Solution*, by Robynne Chutkan. There are also many articles on the Internet – type in the word microbiome and read for hours about this tremendously interesting and important topic. As we learn more about the microbiome, we understand and have more ways to keep ourselves healthy. Remember, health is the number one priority and each day we should strive to be healthier than the day before.

- Dr. Sal

The Importance of Weight Lifting

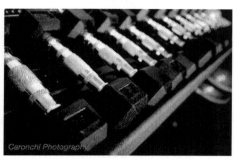

Caronchi Photography

As we get older, one of the things we often notice is that we are not as strong as when we were younger. Our shoulders are not as broad, muscles less defined and the back seems to curve more than it did in the past. Then we go to the doctor for a wellness visit to find out we actually got shorter! We ask, "are you kidding me … I shrunk?" Yes, believe it or not these things do happen as we age. Muscles start to waste away. Bones become less strong. Total body fat and visceral fat (around the internal organs) increases. Metabolism slows, and we gain weight in all the wrong places. Why does this happen and what can we do about it?

The term sarcopenia describes the wasting of muscles and the term osteopenia describes the weakening of the bones. Two reasons for this decline have to do with poor nutrition and physical inactivity, both of which develop in the lives of many Americans as they age. Other reasons include a decrease in testosterone, DHEA, growth hormone and IGF/Insulin-like growth factor. All these hormones are necessary to keep the muscles and bones healthy as we age. Nutritional deficiencies, especially vitamin D, as well as inflammation, also play a major role.

All cells in the body need the proper amounts of healthy proteins, fats, carbohydrates, vitamins, minerals and antioxidants. The standard American diet provides a lot of unhealthy fat, less healthy protein, minimal fiber and many contaminants (pesticides, antibiotics, etc.); and, when the body is not provided with proper nutrition it starts

91

to break down. As the muscles and bones weaken, function declines and we open ourselves to a host of disabling musculoskeletal conditions.

One consequence of aging relates to weakness in the muscles of the lower extremities, associated with an increased risk of falling. This can result in a hip or other bone fracture, the complications of which are often minimized. When you look at what happens to people after they suffer a hip fracture, a large percentage of these folks never get back to normal function and many end up in a nursing home. The take-home message is that hip fractures can be life changing and need to be prevented if possible.

As mentioned above, testosterone and other hormone deficiencies can result in excess fat and weight gain. The added fat creates an enzyme called aromatase which converts some of the remaining testosterone into estrogen; this may result in male breast enlargement. The excess fat also increases the risk of insulin resistance and can cause a pre-diabetic state.

The adipose (fat) cells in the body also produce mediators of inflammation such as C-reactive protein, tumor necrosis factor (TNF) and interleukin 6 (IL-6). The production of these compounds increases inflammation within the body increasing the risk of many chronic illnesses and even cancers.

Vitamin D is an essential nutrient which keeps the muscles and bones healthy. Many people develop vitamin D deficiency due to decreased exposure to the sun, as well as from nutritional deficiencies. In addition to its health effects on the muscles and bones, vitamin D has many other beneficial functions. There are vitamin D receptors in all cells of the body and the beneficial effects are far reaching. Diagnosing vitamin D deficiency is an easy blood test; and, when a person is found to be deficient in vitamin D, the solution is to take supplemental vitamin D3. In addition, it is recommended to get a little sun and add some fortified foods to the diet. Studies have shown that replacement of vitamin D to optimal levels decreases the risk of falling and all its associated complications.

If muscle wasting and bone loss becomes a problem as we age, what can we do about it? We start by optimizing the nutritional value of the foods we eat. We can take in more healthy protein, supplement with glucosamine (which strengthens the cartilage and ligaments supporting the muscles) and get more exercise, especially weight bearing exercises and weight lifting. There is a lot written about how much protein we should eat and the source of the protein. Some of this information is confusing since there is a lot of variability in the recommended amounts, even from the so-called experts in this field. From the research I have done in this area, it seems that the healthy amount is around 1 gram per kilogram of body weight. For a typical man weighing 170 lbs. (77 kg), the requirement for protein would then be 77 grams per day. It is important to understand that excess protein is harmful as it creates a condition called acidosis in the blood; and, when the blood is acidic, it has to be neutralized. As it turns out, the neutralizing factor is calcium which is leached out of the bones. This all leads to weaker bones (osteoporosis) and an increased risk of fractures as well as calcium kidney stones. The individual suffering from sarcopenia (muscle wasting) might require more protein. The amount should be determined by the person's physician in combination with a nutritionist or naturopathic specialist.

Hormone replacement therapy might also be part of the treatment regimen for a person suffering from sarcopenia, osteopenia (weak bones) or osteoporosis (weak bones at risk for fracture). The levels of hormones are measured using blood, saliva and urine tests. Once the levels are known, the physician can prescribe the proper amounts of each specific hormone needed. The best way to replace hormones is with natural, bio-identical hormones rather than with synthetic hormones. Many pharmacies make (compound) the specific dose of bio-identical hormones needed for each individual. Studies have shown bio-identical hormones have fewer side effects since they are the same type of hormones which the body naturally makes. Testosterone can be replaced as a gel, cream, injection or pellets which are placed under the skin and last for a few months. Not only does testosterone replacement to an optimal level help the muscles and bones, studies have shown benefits in relation to depression, overall energy, mood, vitality and sexuality. Replacement of hormones to optimal levels makes a person feel young again!

Finally, in relation to weight lifting, I cannot over emphasize the benefits. For a person who has not been regularly weight lifting, I recommend he/she get a trainer to help design a weight-lifting program. It is most important to learn how to lift weights (or how to use resistance machines) in order to avoid injury. The exercise specialist will determine the proper amount of weight to use initially and how to progress as one gets stronger. This teaching and supervision is vital to the success of any weight-lifting program.

In summary, a comprehensive action plan for improving the strength of the muscles and bones includes: a healthy eating program, weight-lifting exercises, hormone replacement if deficient, stress management to decrease cortisol levels since elevated cortisol increase fat and weight. Quality sleep — growth hormone is made at night during sleep and growth hormone is necessary to rebuild skeletal muscle and vitamin or mineral supplements when necessary. Education is essential to understand and combat the consequences of aging. Two fitness magazines I have found helpful are *FitNation* and *On Fitness*. They both contain great information about exercise, nutrition and general ways to stay healthy and grow older with vitality.

My recommendation for the reader is to work with your primary care physician, exercise specialist, naturopathic physician and nutritionist to design a program that is best for you; then, go out and hit the weights. Your muscles and bones will thank you for it!

- Dr. Sal

Quality and Longevity are Both Important

Most people want to live long lives yet, I wonder sometimes which is more important…quality or the years lived. Many people say they would rather have fewer years as long as they can live the way they want to. In many of these cases, the person is really saying I am okay abusing my health; it makes me feel good and I am okay sacrificing some years for pleasure. This I believe is faulty thinking; we can have pleasure, enjoy a quality life and also live to become many years old.

When we focus on longevity, there are many things we can do to expand life; and, in the process improve the quality of our lives. There are chemicals in many plants and herbs that have been shown to slow the aging process that I will expand on below. It is important to remember that all cellular processes within the body are dependent on the production of ATP energy.

ATP is produced in the mitochondria. These are areas within all cells that make energy. The single most important aspect of health, degenerative disease and aging is the optimal function of the mitochondria. In turn, this is dependent on the availability of macronutrients (proteins, carbohydrates and fats) and micronutrients (vitamins, minerals and antioxidants).

From a broad perspective, it is well known that vitamin and/or mineral deficiency results in age-related diseases and shortens the lifespan. We are constantly bombarded with chemicals, radiation and other toxins which damage the DNA (our genes); and, when we are deficient in vitamins, minerals or antioxidants, the body is less able to repair itself and thus aging advances. Zinc deficiency is a perfect example. When we are low in zinc, the ability to repair cellular damage is decreased.

95

Another essential chemical is omega-3 fat which is found in fish, fish oil, flaxseed and walnuts. It has been shown to have beneficial effects to decrease inflammation, decrease oxidation (rusting of the cells) and strengthen the immune system.

The b-complex vitamins are essential for the proper function of the mitochondria. Niacin, riboflavin and thiamine are all needed to supply essential chemicals to the mitochondria which allows for the production of cellular ATP energy. The mitochondria also need a proper supply of fatty acids and oxygen. Metabolism of fatty acids within the mitochondria depends on thyroid hormone, testosterone, cortisone, human growth hormone and DHEA. Folic acid and vitamin B12 are also needed. You can see how optimal nutrition plays a major role in allowing the body to function. The macro and micronutrients allow for chemical reactions to occur in the cells and this is what actually keeps us alive and well.

In addition to the above, there are many other nutritional supplements and medications known to increase longevity including Metformin, statins, Resveratrol, coenzyme Q10, vitamins C&D, carnosine and DHEA.

Metformin is the most common medication used in the treatment of diabetes. It lowers the absorption of glucose from the GI tract, decreases the production of glucose from the liver and improves the cells' sensitivity to insulin. It also has a positive effect on the metabolism of fats.

Statin medications, such as Lipitor and Crestor, are used for the treatment of elevated cholesterol. When the total cholesterol level is from 182-202, the risk of death from heart disease is 29% higher. When the cholesterol level is above 245, the risk is much greater. In addition to the total cholesterol, when LDL (the bad cholesterol) is high, the risk of heart disease is magnified. Statins are known to decrease total and LDL cholesterol, help stabilize arterial plaque and help repair DNA damage. It is important to realize no medication is without side effects; statins are known to slightly increase the risk of muscle and kidney problems, increase the risk of diabetes and possibly dementia.

Coenzyme Q10 is a fat-soluble vitamin which functions to help produce ATP energy within the mitochondria. It also functions as an anti-oxidant and regenerates other antioxidants which decrease the oxidation (rusting) of LDL cholesterol particles. When LDL becomes oxidized, it is more likely to cause damage to the inner lining of the arteries, known as hardening of the arteries/arteriosclerosis. When the blood level of CoQ 10 is lower than it should be, there is a greater risk of cardiovascular disease, Alzheimer's dementia, diabetes and other neurodegenerative (brain injuring) disorders.

Vitamin C is another essential anti-oxidant. Over the years, humans have lost the ability to make vitamin C therefore it needs to be supplied in the diet. Vitamin C is essential to maintain the health of collagen (the connective tissue below the skin), to decrease the risk of cataracts; it is helpful in people with high blood pressure and heart disease. It might also be helpful for cancer protection.

I have written about the benefits of vitamin D in many previous *News-Press* articles. When most people think of vitamin D, they think you need this for only bone health yet, it is known that vitamin D affects 60 genes and has hundreds of benefits. It helps to decrease the risk of cardiovascular disease, autoimmune disease (when the body makes antibodies which attack itself), as well as neurodegenerative diseases such as multiple sclerosis, Parkinson's and Alzheimer's.

Resveratrol is a chemical found in the skin of red grapes which functions as an anti-oxidant and an activator of sirtuins, an anti-aging protein. Resveratrol enhances the enzyme which produces nitric oxide keeping the blood vessels dilated so blood can move easily. It decreases the oxidation of LDL and helps maintain normal blood glucose/sugar levels.

Carnosine is a chemical which decreases cross-linking (attachment) between sugar molecules and proteins in the body. When a person has too much glucose/sugar in the blood, the glucose molecule attaches to proteins causing the proteins to malfunction. This condition is seen in diabetes, Alzheimer's and many other illnesses. Carnosine has been shown to decrease this abnormal linkage and decrease the risk of these illnesses. It has also been shown to decrease the attachment of glucose to LDL. When glucose attaches to the LDL cholesterol particle, it makes the person more susceptible to arteriosclerosis/hardening of the arteries.

Lastly, DHEA is a pro-hormone and precursor of testosterone and estrogen. As I have mentioned in many other News-Press articles, we cannot age gracefully and fitfully without normal levels of the many hormones which we make so well when we are young. DHEA helps replace these hormones with the goal of getting them back to youthful levels. Underscore the word youthful, since the goal is to regain hormone levels which make us physiologically younger. Supplementation of DHEA helps with this.

Other things that keep us young include exercise, healthy nutrition, avoiding toxins, stress management and getting quality sleep. These are all part of an action plan for healthy living.

In summary, staying young takes work; yet, as can be seen from the above, there are many things we can do to keep our youthful vitality, slow the aging process and live longer. Talk with your physician or health care providers about what you have learned from this article and decide if any of these supplements might be helpful. Then get out and do some exercise! before.

- Dr. Sal

Protect the Brain

When it comes to brain function, it is well known that aging is one of the major risk factors for loss of function. Other risk factors include exposure to toxins (in the air, food, water sources, prescription medications, illegal drugs, cigarette smoke, etc.); also, nutritional deficiencies, hormone imbalance, traumatic brain injury, strokes, recurrent seizures and gut-brain interactions. While this list is not all-inclusive, it illustrates the point that many things affect brain function; therefore, we must do all we can to minimize this decline if we are to live a long, quality life.

In most cases, decreased cognitive function occurs slowly over time. Initially, a person might experience intermittent recall problems such as lost keys, then mild cognitive impairment (MCI) becomes more problematic as it interferes with the activities of daily living. Individuals diagnosed with MCI are at risk for Alzheimer's dementia (AD) and should be counseled on how to slow the progression and reverse it, if possible. Unfortunately, clinical research shows that current medications for the treatment of AD are very ineffective.

Research has shown that exposure to herbicides and pesticides increase the risk and incidence of the most common neurodegenerative disorders such as Parkinson's, Alzheimer's and multiple sclerosis. These chemicals are toxic to the brain and have been proven to be significantly harmful to adults as well as children.

Another toxic substance to the brain is sugar. In some of the medical literature, Alzheimer's is now being called type-3 diabetes. This occurs because the glucose (sugar) molecule attaches to proteins in the brain changing their shape and ultimately the function of these proteins. I have discussed this problem in previous *News-Press* articles and have referred to Advanced Glycation End products (AGEs). If a person has diabetes and is concerned, as they should be, about the risk for Alzheimer's dementia, they should focus on eating a low-carbohydrate diet including healthy fats (avocado, walnuts, flax seeds, fish and fish oil) to protect the brain. Avoiding as many toxins as possible must be part of the action plan to maintain a healthy brain. Other ways to keep the brain healthy include exercise, calorie restriction, hormone balance, anti-oxidant foods and an anti-inflammatory diet. Exercise improves blood flow to the brain. Calorie restriction decreases the toxic load coming from food. Antioxidants are protective to the cells. Hormones decline with age and clinical research proves that supplementing bio-identical hormones back to youthful levels is helpful for the brain and the entire body.

When we think about foods and other things that feed the brain, we know that B- complex vitamins and minerals, such as magnesium and thyroid hormone, are all necessary for brain health. Brain function at the cellular level is no different than cellular function in any other area of the body. It all comes down to chemistry. The cells in the entire body require macronutrients (healthy proteins, fats and carbohydrates), micro nutrients (vitamins and minerals) and antioxidants to function properly. This is the reason we eat nutritious foods and why we take vitamins and supplements.

I have written and lectured on the importance of knowing if your vitamin, mineral and anti-oxidant levels are at healthful levels. In my practice, I use a micro-nutrient test to measure the levels of these essential chemicals. When I lecture, I ask the audience if they understand the function of vitamins. Since most people take them, it is important to understand what they do in the body. The function of vitamins and minerals is to allow chemical reactions to occur. Cellular functions all have to do with chemistry. We must supply the cells with all the essential vitamins, minerals and antioxidants they need to do their job. When we become deficient in any of these essential nutrients, the cells suffer; this is when the body begins to break down,

100

chronic illnesses start to occur and the person is at increased risk of cancer and rapid aging.

We know that inflammation is the common denominator for most chronic illnesses, including most of the neurodegenerative diseases mentioned above. The standard American meal (animal products such as meat and dairy) causes inflammation within the body and brain therefore, the nutritional focus should be on replacing inflammatory foods with nutrients that support healthy brain and body function. Vegetables contain phytonutrients which support total body wellness. Calorie-per-calorie they also provide healthier protein; and, when selecting organic produce, exposes a person to less herbicides and pesticides. When deciding which vegetables and fruits to purchase organically, it is easy to understand that vegetables and fruits with thin skin allow more herbicides and pesticides to get into the deeper layers and should be purchased as organic. When the label on these items starts with the number nine, you know that the product is organic. Labels starting with the number four are conventionally grown and are exposed to traditional herbicides and pesticides; while those starting with the number eight are genetically modified (GMO) foods and should be avoided.

As I have recommended many times in the past, get your vitamins, minerals and antioxidants from the foods you eat. Supplementation is necessary when you eat a healthy diet and still have lower than acceptable levels. When it comes to supplements to help maintain a healthy brain, there are several including vitamin B2 (riboflavin), needed for the metabolism of fats and glucose; 1-creatine, needed for the mitochondria to make energy (ATP); carnitine which shuttles fats into the mitochondria (the parts of the cell that make energy), Co Q-10, an anti-oxidant that protects the cells from rusting and wearing out, omega-3 fatty acids (EPA & DHA) necessary to maintain the health of all cell membranes, and rhodiola, a plant product that helps the cells make energy. I refer the reader to a naturopathic specialist, an integrative medicine physician or a nutritionist/dietician for more direction regarding healthy supplements.

In addition to the above, another organ which we must protect in order to maintain a healthy brain is the gut, the gastrointestinal tract. I have written about the gut-brain connection many times in the past and talked about it extensively. There is a direct and indirect connection between the gut and the brain; when the gut is not healthy, the brain cannot be maximally healthy. For the reader who wants to learn more about this topic, please read, *Gut feelings: the biology of gut-brain communication in Nature Review* and also read, *The Microbiome Solution*, by Dr. Robynne Chutkan.

We know what we eat and drink significantly influences the health of all organs and every cell in the body. It is most important to make the right choices for what we put into and what we do not allow access to our body. When you do this for the majority of meals that you eat, you will undoubtedly live a longer and higher quality life. So...enjoy healthy food and enjoy a healthy life!

- Dr. Sal

Your Medical Community Rallies Around Food

In the past we held the annual *Food is Medicine* (FIM) meeting and doubled the number of health care providers attending! The FIM committee was started because we became more aware that traditional medicine was becoming a branch of the pharmaceutical industry, more people were developing chronic illnesses and we realized we are losing the war against cancer. As people were becoming overweight and developing more diabetes and Alzheimer's, we looked for the common denominator and found it in food.

At the start of this year's FIM meeting, I showed the video, *Rewind the Future*, which depicts a 32-year old obese male being wheeled into the emergency room unconscious from a heart attack. The ER doctors ask, "How does this happen?" The video then rewinds this man's life to show it is obvious that all of his days are centered on an obsession with eating food, mostly unhealthy food. Unfortunately, his parents fed into the problem, as the mother states by giving him fast-food French fries to keep him quiet. At an early age, he develops an obsession and addiction to junk food; it is no wonder that by 32-years of age he develops a heart attack.

As a society, we have placed food at the center of our lives; over the past 50 years we have produced more unhealthy food, relied more on pills to cure our ills and have become an extremely sedentary society — all contributing to the dismal state of health of the population. Our country ranks far behind most other developed countries in health parameters, despite spending twice what every other developed country spends on health care. Our health care system has become a sick care system. It no longer focuses on wellness, instead must focus on taking care of people with chronic illness and

103

cancer. We need to go back to a system that promotes health and wellness; again, food is at the core of this solution — this time the emphasis is on HEALTHY FOOD!

After we watched the video, I reiterated that food either leads us down the road to chronic illness and cancer or it leads us down the road to a healthy life where we are able to grow older gracefully and fitfully, rather than simply growing old.

The vision of the FIM committee is to incorporate the use of healthy food into mainstream medical care for the prevention of illness and the mission is to disseminate up-to-date, scientific, evidence-based recommendations regarding the benefits of nutrition on health. The goal is to infuse this information into mainstream medical care so each patient-physician interaction involves a discussion about the benefits of healthy eating.

Since the last FIM meeting a year ago, we developed a flyer which can be placed in the doctors' exam rooms to remind patients to "Ask about Food is Medicine!" The committee developed this flyer to stimulate the discussion knowing that most people need to improve their diet. The flyer describes an Optimal Nutrition Approach which we believe is eating a variety of nutrient rich, whole foods, including several servings of colorful vegetables per day, a few servings of fruits, whole grains, nuts, beans and other lean proteins which supply the body what is needed for optimal health. This nutrition plan also recommends avoiding highly processed foods and concentrated sugary drinks while encouraging regular physical activity.

In addition, we developed a *Healthy Plate* flyer which is a picture of a food plate with proper proportions of vegetables, fruits, whole grains and healthy proteins. It contains wording detailing serving number or size, specific proteins to eat for maintaining good health, explains that every tablespoon of oil contains 120 calories, recommends drinking lots of water and staying active. This Healthy Plate is a great visual to use with my patients helping them understand how to develop healthy eating habits. With this information, we all can eat healthy at home and when we eat out. It gives us the knowledge to create our own healthy plate and puts us on the road to healthy living and a healthy life.

At this meeting we also discussed the PlantPure Nation Jumpstart program and the CHIP program. These are two very helpful nutrition programs which teach people how to eat healthy. Jumpstart is a ten-day in-home healthy nutrition program; the CHIP (Complete Health Improvement) program is a nine-week in-class nutrition program with a focus on how to shop, cook and eat healthy foods.

As I write this article and think about this third annual *Food is Medicine* meeting, I am very proud of the team we have built and how passionate people are dedicated to promoting another way of life helping people become and stay healthy. As I say in all my presentations, "health is the number one priority" — we must cherish it every day! When we lose our good health, all else fails. When we lose our health, we spend much time, money and effort to get it back. The message is, "Don't lose it in the first place then you won't have to worry about getting it back!" Chronic disease and cancers are avoidable. Most chronic disease and many of the common cancers are due to lifestyle and not genetics. Growing older does not mean we have to get old with disease. We are meant to grow older with vitality; and, as is shown in those areas of the world where people live into their 100s, our DNA has been designed to live that long — why not take advantage of it?

- Dr. Sal

Fighting For Air

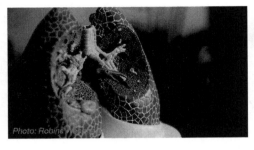

Photo: Robine

My father passed away in 2010 after about 15 years with emphysema. He spent much of the last year of life in and out of the hospital and unfortunately, he died suddenly in the hospital, all alone. My brother, mother and I visited with him the afternoon of his death. While at my mother's house, we received a call from the hospital saying he had passed away. What was amazing was we left him in good spirits sitting aside the hospital bed, looking better than he had in a long time. He gave us the thumbs up as we left and smiled.

Fighting for air is what happens when a person smokes for a long period of time. This is what may happen to many of the current smokers who are now switching to vapor/e-cigarettes. The problem with these types of inhaled devices is they are not regulated. When I sit in my car at a red light and look at folks in other cars, often someone is smoking a vapor cigarette. What strikes me is the depth of their inhalations, how long they keep this smoky chemical in their lungs and the amount of smoke that comes out when they exhale. I believe they are able to inhale much deeper and for a longer time because the smoke from these vapor cigarettes is not hot like a traditional cigarette. These are the reasons we will see people fighting for air after using these devices for extended periods. Over the next 10-20 years we are going to see a number of new lung problems, possibly even new types of lung cancers.

There are so many different medical problems we deal with today, many of which are essentially man-made. Even many of the common cancers are known to be at least partially due to lifestyle behaviors. Think also about the number of autoimmune diseases which now number over 100! These are diseases where the body actually attacks itself. Many of these diseases have inflammation as the common denominator. When the body is inflamed, disease and cancer occur. Inflammation comes from many of the foods people eat (the standard American diet), from drinks we consume, from radiation, drugs, heavy metals, toxins like pesticides and herbicides.

Emphysema, lung cancer, chronic bronchitis, asthma and autoimmune lung diseases may pale in comparison to new lung problems which might come about in the years to come. How will we treat and reverse these new illnesses? I realize all this is speculation, but shouldn't we err on the side of caution? Shouldn't we do all we can to keep our lungs and our bodies healthy?

The American Lung Association sponsors an annual Fight for Air Climb. This is an event where people walk or run up 31 stories of the Oasis Tower in Fort Myers, Florida in honor of someone who is dealing with a lung disease or someone who has passed from one. I do this in honor of my father with my daughter, Isabella.

Preventive health care and wellness is what I am passionate about. People should avoid disease rather than trying to treat and reverse it. The focus is to stay well by living healthy lives, not smoking any kind of cigarette, eating nutritious food and by exercising regularly.

- Dr. Sal

Is Your Medicine Cabinet Making You Sick?

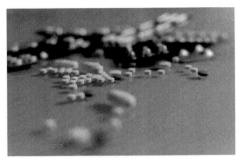

A statement about the current condition of health care caught my attention when the author described his feeling that the health care industry has become a branch of the pharmaceutical industry. After watching the multitude of television ads for drugs, perhaps his assessment is not far off the mark.

Certainly, many health problems today are initially treated with medications. We treat hypertension (elevated blood pressure) and high cholesterol. We use medication to lower the pressure and cholesterol level before we find and eliminate the cause. We know that most chronic illnesses are related to unhealthy lifestyle behaviors and by adjusting to a healthier lifestyle, these problems are resolved. This is especially the case with cardiovascular disease. For more information about this, read Reversing Heart Disease, by Dr. Caldwell Esselstyn. The same can be said of diabetes including Dr. Joel Furhman's book, The End of Diabetes.

Recently I expressed my frustration with the television commercial for an acid-lowering medication showing the actor eating very unhealthy food causing his heartburn. Instead of the commercial advising us not to eat the unhealthy food, the actor recommends "eat what you want" and then "take this pill" and the symptoms will be resolved. We create the problem we then need to treat. We should eliminate the offending foods to solve the problem.

A better solution to many health problems can be found in your kitchen. When you look in your refrigerator, you hopefully will find vegetables, fruits and other healthy foods that contain chemicals keeping us healthy. For example, broccoli and other cruciferous vegetables contain sulforaphane, a chemical known to decrease the risk of breast and other cancers. Carrots contain vitamin A which helps keep the eyes healthy; vitamin A is also a good antioxidant which decreases the risk of vascular disease and other chronic health problems.

When the pantry contains herbs and spices, these are added to the anti-cancer arsenal. Curcumin (turmeric) is a perfect example; this spice should be added to as many dishes as possible since it is a strong anti-cancer substance. Most of the vitamins, minerals and antioxidants we need to stay healthy should come from the foods we eat. If a supplement is needed, it is important to have a blood test to ascertain what specific vitamin or mineral you are deficient in; then take a good quality supplement along with healthy, nutritious meals.

Coenzyme-Q (Co Q) is another supplement required for the production of energy (ATP) and is a powerful antioxidant. Rich dietary sources include almonds, ocean salmon, sardines, spinach and certain meats. The immune cells in the body divide more rapidly than most other cells and are in constant need of repair/maintenance and these functions require energy; therefore, Co Q is an important supplement for the immune system. We know that the level decreases as we age; therefore, if we are not getting enough from the diet, we should take a supplement. Levels of Co Q also decrease with certain medications such as statins used to lower cholesterol. Co Q is highly concentrated in the heart, brain and muscles. These are all organs requiring a lot of energy and we do not want to fall short on this vital substance.

Vitamin D3 acts more like a hormone than a vitamin. It has many functions within the body and is essential for healthy aging. We can make D3 from sunlight, from fatty fish, fortified foods and vitamin supplements. In addition to keeping our bones healthy, vitamin D also maintains the health of the immune system, keeps the nerves and

109

muscles healthy and decreases inflammation within the body. It also has a role in the function of genes which make proteins that control cell growth.

Cinnamon is another healthy spice which can be added to oatmeal along with fresh berries and almond milk for a great morning breakfast. When preparing that delicious soup for lunch or dinner, add some turmeric. Parsley, basil and oregano should be part of your anti-cancer meal plan. Adding pepper to meals has been reported in a study from the University of Michigan to lower the risk of breast cancer, especially when combined with turmeric.

With your new knowledge, I hope you will see your kitchen and medicine cabinet in a new light. Preferably, your medicine cabinet will look bare — the goal is to take as few medications as possible. Your refrigerator, pantry and kitchen cabinets will be loaded with healthy foods. There are times when prescription medications are necessary. Plan on reaching for natural disease fighting foods first, as well as creating a healthy lifestyle, before reaching for the pills.

- Dr. Sal

Age Related Macular Degeneration (AMD)

Age-Related Macular Degeneration (AMD) is the leading cause of irreversible blindness in the U.S. among people 50 years and older. The earliest reports of this problem date back to 1874 when it was termed symmetric, central choroido-retinal disease occurring in senile persons. Currently, there are about eight million people living with AMD; this number is projected to increase 50% by 2020.

The macula is that part of the retina (the back of the eye) responsible for central visual acuity allowing a person to see fine details, read and recognize faces. Blood supply to the macula and this portion of the retina comes from behind the eye. As we age, debris collects in this area decreasing the blood and nutrient supply to the eye. When an ophthalmologist examines the back of the eye, they can see what are called drusen which represent focal deposits of a cellular material (debris) which over time decreases visual acuity. The diagnosis relies on the presence of drusen irrespective of the visual acuity. In the early stage of AMD, the visual loss is minimal; as more drusen develop, the visual loss becomes apparent and problematic.

There are two forms of AMD characterized as dry and wet. The dry form is clinically termed geographic atrophy which represents the gradual breakdown of light-sensitive cells in the macula that send visual information to the brain. The wet form is called neovascular AMD since abnormal blood vessels grow under the macula. These vessels can leak fluid and blood leading to swelling (edema) and damage to the macula. Unlike the more gradual loss of vision which occurs with dry AMD, the loss of vision with the wet form can be rapid and severe. It is possible to have both forms of dry and wet AMD in the same eye.

111

Risk factors for AMD include cigarette smoking, Caucasian ethnicity and those with a family history or a genetic susceptibility. At last count, researchers have identified about 20 gene defects which increase the susceptibility of AMD yet there is not one gene defect which unequivocally makes the diagnosis by a dilated eye examination. Since there are few symptoms in the early stage of ADM, it is important to have the eyes examined annually.

Other lifestyle behaviors which increase the risk for AMD include poor nutrition, a sedentary lifestyle and any factor which increases the blood pressure. These risk factors can be discussed during a wellness examination, allowing the individual and the physician to create an action plan to deal with the risk factors.

It is helpful to understand that not everyone with early AMD goes on to develop late AMD. For those with early AMD in one eye, about 5% will develop late AMD within 10 years. For those with early AMD in both eyes, about 14% will go on to advanced disease within 10 years.

Because there is no treatment for early AMD, prevention is essential. It is known that AMD occurs less often in those who exercise, eat lots of green, leafy vegetables and do not smoke. For those with intermediate stage AMD, research has shown that high-dose vitamins and minerals can slow the progression of the disease.

The first Age-Related Eye Disease Study (AREDS) trial showed that a combination of vitamin C, vitamin E, beta-carotene, zinc and copper can reduce the risk of late AMD by 25%. The second AREDS showed that adding lutein and zeaxanthin or omega 3 fatty acids to the original formulation added no additional benefit; however, when they removed the beta-carotene and added a 5:1 ratio of lutein and zeaxanthin, the risk of late stage AMD decreased further. A number of manufacturers offer nutritional supplements based on the results of the AREDS studies. The reader can refer to these studies for the doses of the specific nutritional supplements and should consult with an ophthalmologist before starting any supplements or medications to help with eye disease.

One of the immediate things a person can do to improve eye health, as well as total body health, is to quit smoking all kinds of cigarettes, even vapor/e-cigarettes. Tobacco smoke decreases blood flow to all areas of the body; by stopping this unhealthy behavior, an individual lowers his/her risk for not only AMD but also most chronic lung diseases and many cancers including lung, bladder and colon.

For those with advanced AMD, there are a number of procedures an ophthalmologist can perform in an attempt to slow the progression and hopefully stop further vision loss. These include injections, photodynamic therapy and laser surgery. The injections are used to slow the development of new blood vessels (neovascularization). In this form of advanced AMD (neovascular AMD) a protein called VEGF (vascular endothelial growth factor) is secreted into the eye. By blocking this protein by administering an Anti-VEGF drug, the growth of new blood vessels in the area of the macula can be slowed.

Photodynamic therapy involves the administration of a medication which is injected into a vein of the arm then travels to the eye and is absorbed by new blood vessels. The eye specialist then shines a laser beam into the eye to activate the drug which closes off the new blood vessels while sparing normal blood vessels.

Laser therapy involves the use of a hot laser to close off the abnormally growing blood vessels around the area of the macula. Laser therapy can destroy surrounding healthy tissue and result in a small blind spot. If you have advanced AMD, please discuss these options with your eye specialist.

Most readers, I am sure, will agree that vision holds a special place in a person's life and we need to do all we can to keep our eyes healthy. We can do this by not smoking, exercising regularly, eating lots of colorful vegetables, taking vitamins and/or supplements when necessary; and, by visiting with an eye specialist annually to be sure there are no signs of early AMD. For more information about eye disease, I refer the reader to the American Academy of Ophthalmology online at aao.org.

- Dr. Sal

How Do Plants Protect Themselves From Disease?

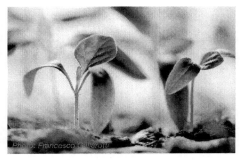

Photo: Francesco Villaretti

In the last five years, I have read hundreds of clinical research reports about the health benefits of plants and have looked into how plants themselves actually avoid disease. The answer relates to the chemicals that plants produce, which in essence protect the plants from disease.

Let's review the chemical resveratrol which is found in the skin of red grapes. Resveratrol is what is called a phytoalexin, a naturally occurring chemical within plants which is part of the plants' defense mechanism against environmental challenges such as microbial infections from bacteria, viruses and fungi. In addition to their antibacterial, antiviral and antifungal properties, these beneficial chemicals within plants act as antioxidants which essentially keep the cells within plants from rusting.

Resveratrol is also a potent phytoestrogen, a plant estrogen which is thought to block the harmful effects of more powerful estrogens, thereby decreasing the risk of breast and other GYN cancers.

Resveratrol in some studies appears to be an indirect activator of the sirtuin genes which are longevity genes. These genes also act as calorie restriction mimetics, meaning they act in a similar fashion to calorie restriction (CR). Clinical research studies have shown that reducing the calories we eat results in a longer lifespan. The explanation is at least partially related to a decrease in toxins that results from simply eating less food. Most processed foods are

115

contaminated with chemicals and other harmful substances. If we eat less calories (less food), we subject our body to less toxic exposure and live longer! Resveratrol has been shown in some studies to mimic the effects of calorie restriction by indirectly turning on sirtuin genes, resulting in a longer lifespan — how cool is that!

Resveratrol also contains what are called MMP inhibitors which basically inhibit the breakdown of collagen (the parts of the skin which keep it looking youthful). This mechanism makes resveratrol attractive as a skin anti-aging substance; yet, it might also be helpful in cancer treatment since it is known that cancer cells spread by breaking down collagen.

Resveratrol appears to have protective effects against hardening of the arteries (arteriosclerosis) by regulating nitric oxide (NO). Nitric oxide is the chemical produced by the cells lining the inner portion of blood vessels causing vasodilatation. Nitric oxide improves blood circulation. Resveratrol also decreases the production of another chemical called endothelin, known to cause plaque formation in the walls of arteries. By decreasing the production of endothelin, resveratrol decreases arteriosclerosis/ hardening of the arteries. This helps to lower blood pressure, another beneficial effect on the cardiovascular system. Resveratrol decreases the stickiness of platelets, blood clotting, the risk of strokes and heart attacks. This probably explains why people who drink red wine have a lower risk of heart attacks and strokes.

Quercetin is another chemical found in plants (a plant flavonoid) with multiple beneficial effects, including antioxidant and antihistamine properties. This chemical has been associated with a lower risk of cardiovascular disease and cancer. Ellagic acid is a naturally occurring phenol antioxidant found in most berries, pecans, walnuts and grapes. It is thought to be helpful to decrease the risk of cancer by decreasing the ability of carcinogens (cancer causing substances) to bind to DNA. We know that cancer causing chemicals called nitrosamines are found in grilled meats as well as processed lunch meats. When the cells of our body become exposed to these carcinogens, the DNA (genetic material) can become disrupted leading to the production of cancer cells. With this explanation we can understand why eating berries and nuts is so beneficial. If we can eat and enjoy these foods and they help us to avoid cancer, why would we not eat them on a regular basis?

What has been described above is the new field of nutrigenomics — the effects of nutrition on genes and how chemicals within vegetables, fruits and other foods we eat either lead to better health or lead to chronic disease and cancer. Other examples are found in green tea which contains the chemical ECGC, genistein which is found in soy, lycopene in tomatoes and curcumin found in the Indian spice, turmeric. In addition to food, other epigenetic factors (environmental or lifestyle factors which affect our genes) include physical activity, emotional status, toxins within our environment and many inherited factors. Cancer prevention occurs not only in relation to the number of phytonutrients (plant chemical nutrients as described above) we consume daily but also by what we are exposed to on a daily basis. If our lifestyle behaviors are unhealthy and the environment we live in is toxic, we are more likely to suffer from chronic disease and cancer.

There has been a rise in the number of autoimmune diseases over the last century. We now have over 100 known autoimmune diseases such as rheumatoid arthritis, lupus, multiple sclerosis, thyroid disease, colitis — the list goes on. We need to understand that our exposures affect our health in a major way; and, that we have more control over this than we believe. Our lifestyle can indeed affect our genes. Our genetic makeup at birth is not necessarily our destiny. By making the right choices in relation to what we eat, how we exercise, how we sleep and manage our stress, we can keep cancer genes turned off and healthy genes turned on.

Our actions need to be intentional and we should set a goal to move closer and closer to a healthier lifestyle each day. None of us are perfect in our behaviors and getting to a healthier lifestyle is a journey. Each day we can do a little more to move us down the road to better health. When we fall off the wagon, we simply need to get back on and continue with positive movement forward. Speak encouraging words to yourself and congratulate yourself for the positive changes you make in your life. Do the same for friends and family who work on a regular basis to get healthier. Hang out with like-minded people who cherish their health and support one another. Read as much as you can about healthy living and make this a part of your everyday life. ***Make Health Last*** is the You Tube video I recommend people watch; and, as I tell my patients and those who attend my public presentations, make health last by making health first — your first and number one priority!

Awesome Days Result in Better Health

It was an awesome day. The American Lung Association hosts an annual stair climb competition to raise awareness and research dollars for lung diseases. This year's event was different since I was able to climb the 553 steps with my daughter in honor of my father who passed away in 2010 from emphysema. As she has done many times, Bella amazed me with her physical stamina. We climbed the 31 flights in 5 minutes and 57 seconds! This is amazing to me since Bella had open-heart surgery when she was 2 years old and now is able to do more than most children her age and older.

Next, I joined Dr. Brian Taschner, Dr. Jose Colon and Dr. Sebastian Klisiewicz for a four-hour presentation where we all spoke on how the standard American diet creates disease and disability; and, how truly nutritious food creates health, vitality and longevity. Dr. Taschner focused on how nutrition relates to cardiovascular disease. Dr. Colon spoke not only about sleep as it relates to health, but how nutrition affects the mitochondria (the powerhouse of the cells). Dr. Klisiewicz presented many research reports on how food affects musculoskeletal health and various rheumatologic disorders. I finished the morning reviewing dozens of research studies on the benefits of spices, micronutrients and lifestyle factors in the generation of health and avoidance of disease.

The goal was to share with the audience the science of nutrition and increase awareness among health care professionals of the vital role nutrition has in traditional health care. We emphasized that nutrition should be the starting point for all treatment plans as well as the foundation for any preventive health care program. The importance of exercise and how physical activity has been proven to decrease the risk not only of cardiovascular disease but also Alzheimer's, obesity, diabetes, depression and so many other chronic illnesses as well as the foundation for any preventive health care program. I mentioned to the attendees that much of the information presented at this conference has been around for many years; yet for some reason(s), much of this objective, clinical, research supported data has been ignored. We are now on a journey to spread the word on nutrition and make it clear that a discussion about healthy eating needs to happen in the exam rooms, while sharing meals with our family, when our children take meals at school and outside the home.

Research studies and anecdotal reports consistently reinforce the need to place nutrition at the top of the list of daily priorities. When we fuel our body with healthy, nutritious food and drink, we are able to accomplish all other priorities. When we do the opposite, many of our priorities fail since we lack energy, our brains are not maximally functional, our immune system is not able to protect us from infection as optimally as it should; and, we become susceptible to chronic disease, cancer and even early death.

Obviously, the lesson is to eat healthy food every day and life is good! Attend educational presentations, read and become aware of the things you can do to control your health. It is time to make a strong commitment to nutrition as one of the foundational aspects of a healthy life and understand the importance of quality sleep and other lifestyle behaviors. This presentation was attended by about 65 physicians, dieticians, therapists, other health care providers and some interested folks from the general community. Drs. Taschner, Colon, Klisiewicz and I were very excited to see so many engaged participants – another reason this awesome day resulted in better health!

The last part of my awesome day supports the belief that having fun results in better health. A few months ago, I was asked to be a judge for the Dancing Classrooms program founded by Pierre Dulaine in New York. Dancing Classrooms is a social and emotional development program for fifth grade students, using ballroom dancing as a vehicle to change the lives of the children and their families. I accepted the invitation with a little reservation and nervousness. While I have taken many ballroom dance lessons and even done an amateur competition in the past, I had never judged a competition.

The master of ceremonies, Rodney Lopez, instructed us on how we should judge the dancers. There were eight teams from local elementary schools. They each had dance couples dedicated to a particular dance; we judged meringue, swing, rumba, tango and foxtrot. At the end of the competition, the teams received either a bronze, silver or gold medal. All participants had their medals hung around their neck similar to the Olympics. What a wonderfully, exciting time for all these students who were so happy to be involved in this life changing event.

My healthy living recommendation is to go out and have an awesome day. Get involved in a group exercise program, an educational session and a fun event like a dance competition or even a dance lesson for yourself! Live life to the fullest, enjoy being with other people and, stay well my friends!

- Dr. Sal

Go Red For Women!

Recently I attended the American Heart Association Go Red for Women event at the Hyatt Regency in Bonita Springs and witnessed the hundreds of women and men who attended to raise awareness and money for heart disease research. The sea of women dressed in red and the men with their red ties was a beautiful site.

The keynote speaker was Dr. Marc Braman, past president of the American College of Lifestyle Medicine and current president of the Lifestyle Medicine Foundation. Dr. Braman spoke about the association between heart disease and lifestyle; he helped the audience understand how preventable heart disease is when lifestyle behaviors are applied. He also described the work of Dr. Caldwell Esselstyn who was able to prove that cardiovascular disease is reversible! The overwhelming importance of these last two sentences basically states that heart disease (cardiovascular disease) is preventable and reversible — truly amazing!

We know that heart disease is the number one killer of women in the U.S., taking one life every minute. We also know the risk factors include smoking, high cholesterol, high blood pressure, diabetes and pre-diabetes, obesity, sedentary lifestyle and family history. Similar to men, women with unbalanced hormones, including a low testosterone level have a higher risk of cardiovascular disease. This is because testosterone acts as an anti-inflammatory chemical in the body and brain; when the level is low, there is more inflammation in the body which can manifest as heart disease.

The terms heart disease and cardiovascular disease are used interchangeably. To be more correct, we should use the term cardiovascular disease (CVD) consistently since blood vessel disease in the heart means that a person most likely has it in other areas of the circulation system. Cardiovascular disease is the manifestation of endothelial dysfunction.

Dr. Braman explained the concept of inflammation causing cardiovascular disease. Inflammation is the common denominator for all vascular diseases as well as for certain types of dementia, autoimmune diseases, musculoskeletal disorders and other health problems. One goal in the treatment of CVD is to lower the level of inflammation in the body.

As we age, many areas of the body weaken, and the heart is no exception. There are many things which can be done to slow the deterioration and even reverse the process. Most people know of the benefits of exercise but often use no time as an excuse for not exercising regularly. When designing an action plan to stay healthy and age slowly and fitfully, we must fit exercise into our daily lives. The general recommendation is to have at least 30 minutes of moderately intense exercise on most days of the week; yet, realize that the duration can be shortened if the intensity is increased. Studies show that higher intensity exercise with shorter duration is actually more beneficial for the heart and lungs. The Harvard Alumni study published in 1995 showed a reduced risk of death with high versus moderate or low-intensity exercise. The European Heart Journal reported that high intensity exercise improves peak oxygen uptake. Lastly, the Journal of Applied Physiology in 2009 reported on the effects sprinting (fast running for short periods) versus endurance training (jogging slowly on a treadmill for longer periods of time) had on oxygen uptake, again showed that shorter duration, higher intensity exercises were more beneficial for the heart and lungs.

This information might make one think that many of the current exercise programs result in less than optimal benefit for the cardiopulmonary system. Many research studies do support the concept of higher intensity training; one important thing to keep in mind is that every individual is different and as such, exercise programs must be designed specifically for each individual. The intensity of any exercise program should be progressed slowly. For any individual who has already suffered a heart attack, the exercise program should be designed by his/her cardiologist in conjunction with a professionally educated physical therapist specializing in cardiac rehabilitation. The program usually involves aerobic training (brisk walking, jogging, swimming and biking) in combination with resistance/weight training. Both aspects of an exercise program should be progressively accelerated to achieve maximal benefit. As the person is monitored, the cardiologist and exercise specialist determine when to increase the intensity and how much an increase is appropriate. This should be done for the aerobic exercise as well as the resistance/weight training. The only way to keep the heart, muscles, bones, brain and the entire body healthy, strong and functional is to challenge all parts. When this is done for those with existing CVD under the supervision of a cardiologist and exercise specialists, the results can be amazing. The goal should be to get the individual maximally functional and to reverse the disease process.

Other ways to reverse the disease include decreasing as many risk factors for CVD as possible, designing a healthy eating plan, limiting processed foods especially those laden with saturated fat and sugar, using supplements like CoQ 10 (a supplement which helps the heart make energy) and focusing on health as the number one priority every day. All of these recommendations will help lower the level of inflammation within the body. When cholesterol levels are not in the goal range with lifestyle modification alone, the individual should talk with his/her physician about medications. Treatment should be a combination of risk factor reduction, moving closer each day to a healthier lifestyle, medications when the benefits outweigh the risk of pharmaceuticals and close follow up with health care providers who can effectively treat, reverse and prevent disease.

In his opening statement, Dr. Braman asked who was responsible for fixing the problem of CVD and the answer was — we all are! Each person must be responsible for their health and consistently do a little more each day to become and stay healthy. We need to work in conjunction with a physician and other health care providers to develop an action plan that brings results for all involved. This is a team effort.

I encourage my patients to watch the You Tube video, Make Health Last; it is a sobering presentation of a typical American living the last years of his life in sickness and contrasts this with the last years of life being spent in wellness as a result of living a healthy life. Like life in general, achieving good health is a journey. We travel down this road each day. Sometimes we veer off course but as long as we get back on the healthy road, the end result will be good. The goal is to live the last years of your life in wellness being fit, vital, functional and a productive part of family and community. It is our responsibility to do this and stay on the healthy road — which road will you choose?

- Dr. Sal

Do We Die of Old Age or Lack of Energy?

In preparation for an anti-aging certification examination, I read about some of the theories of aging and one theory is that we age and die because we essentially run out of energy. This concept intrigued me to read more about how energy is produced within our cells and came across an article on AMPK. This compound found in every cell in the body is responsible for maintaining a proper balance of energy.

The fundamental unit of energy within all cells is adenosine triphosphate (ATP). As cells need energy, they use ATP which is converted into adenosine monophosphate (AMP). As the level of AMP increases, it essentially tells the cell it is running out of energy; that is when AMPK/AMP kinase kicks into gear. AMPK has been called the master metabolic switch, allowing cells to maintain a proper level of energy/ATP.

When AMPK is activated, it increases the transport of glucose and fats into the mitochondria, the powerhouse of the cell. Glucose and fats/fatty acids are necessary for the mitochondria to make energy/ATP. Carnitine is another substance involved in this process; it helps glucose and fats get into the mitochondria. Once inside, the glucose and fats are used by the mitochondria to make energy. This process also uses coenzyme Q10 (Co Q10). People who take a statin drug for high cholesterol are also prescribed Co Q10 (which is depleted by the statin drug). Co Q10 is necessary for the cell to make energy.

Many studies have been done to understand the mechanisms involved in cellular energy production; these studies have shown that cells capable of maintaining proper levels of ATP live longer. The studies have also shown that activated AMPK promotes energy release and suppresses energy storage. This means that the organism is more energetic and leaner since glucose and fats are used for energy production and not stored in fat cells, in the liver or in the skeletal muscles. When an organism functions more in the realm of energy storage, it becomes fatter with less energy and a shorter lifespan.

This mechanism brings to mind the American lifestyle. Over the past 50-100 years Americans have become more sedentary, consume more calories, gained more weight and have developed more chronic illness and cancer than any time in history. If we look at the cells of a typical American, we would see less ATP and less activated AMPK since the cells are functioning to store rather than burn energy.

It is clear that when calorie intake is higher, AMPK activation is diminished, less ATP is made and the glucose and fats are then used to store energy as fat under the skin —and even more detrimentally around the vital organs such as the heart, liver and kidneys. Storing fat in this fashion leads to the development of the metabolic syndrome/ metsyn. This syndrome is a combination of elevated blood glucose, triglycerides/fats, blood pressure, waist circumference and low HDL (good cholesterol). Three or more of these metabolic abnormalities is the definition of metsyn and confers a significant risk for cardiovascular and neurodegenerative diseases. The individual is more at risk for heart attacks, strokes, dementia, diabetes, obesity and shortened lifespan.

A common denominator in all these illnesses is inflammation. It is well known that inflammation further suppresses activation of AMPK, resulting in the cells having more difficulty in making the necessary energy. We know that the standard American diet and lifestyle is inflammatory; it has been said that we are eating ourselves to death. This is essentially the SAD truth (the standard American diet)!

The good news is that we can restore AMPK to optimal levels through a combination of healthy nutrition, exercise, supplements, lifestyle behaviors and a prescription medication, Metformin. The reader might recognize Metformin as the most common diabetes medication and it is known that Metformin is a potent activator of AMPK. Interestingly, a study in 2014 showed that diabetics treated with Metformin lived about 15% longer; and, it was explained that this was most likely due to activation of AMPK as well as other mechanisms. This was in contrast to other diabetes medications such as sulfonylureas which are not AMPK activators.

The term gerosuppressor has been used to describe the actions of AMPK, meaning that it suppresses aging. We know that aging is associated with a decline in the number and function of the mitochondria; and, studies have shown that AMPK not only activates ATP production within the mitochondria, it also helps to regenerate mitochondria.

In addition, AMPK stimulates the production and activation of sirtuin genes which are referred to as longevity genes. Research has shown that activation of these genes allows the organism to live longer. AMPK also inhibits one of the master regulators of inflammation called NF-kappa beta. This is another compound within cells which stimulates immune reactions leading to inflammation and dysfunction within cells. Inhibition of NF-kB decreases inflammation and allows the cells to function properly.

AMPK has been shown to extend lifespan in several species by enhancing energy production, by supporting the mitochondria, reducing inflammation and enhancing the immune system. It inhibits the growth of cancer cells, decreasing oxidation of LDL cholesterol, decreasing the production of arterial plaque, by decreasing blood pressure, reducing insulin resistance and decreasing the risk of the metabolic syndrome.

As we age, we must increase our activity levels. While exercising, you use ATP/energy and the higher levels of AMP stimulate the activity of AMPK making more energy. Another is calorie restriction (CR) which has been shown to stimulate the activity of the longevity genes (sirtuin genes). There are also a few supplements which have been shown to increase AMPK activation, namely gynostemma (a traditional Vietnamese herb) and trans-tiliroside, a bioactive compound obtained from the fruit of the rose plant. Gynostemma activates AMPK which then lowers fasting blood glucose as well as the three-month average blood glucose level. When added to traditional diabetes medication, the effect is even more beneficial. Trans-tiliroside increases fat burning and decreases fat storage; it has also been shown to decrease blood pressure and decrease total and LDL cholesterol. The combination of these natural supplements with exercise and calorie restriction results in greater activation of AMPK; increases cellular energy which translates into healthier cells able to function optimally for longevity.

In summary, there are many things we can do to maintain energy as we age and by doing these things, we can age more gracefully, more fitfully and slower. No need to rush the aging process!

- Dr. Sal

Why is Heart Disease the #1 Killer in the U.S.?

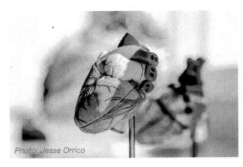
Photo: Jesse Orrico

It has long been known that heart disease is the number one killer in the U.S. Why is this? Before I answer, let me explain that heart disease is a manifestation of vascular disease; and, when arteries are clogged in the heart, they are probably clogged in other arteries. This is a total body vascular disease that we have to deal with comprehensively.

A heart attack or stroke is the end result of years of dysfunction of the endothelium, the inner lining of the arteries. During this process, the arteries go from being normal to being occluded (producing a heart attack or a stroke) over years and possibly decades. There are many things that injure the arteries; they respond by creating inflammation, oxidative stress and abnormal immune responses. Inflammation is the hallmark of endothelial dysfunction where the inner lining of the arteries starts to develop early plaque. As the injury and inflammation continue, plaque increases. The covering of the plaque called the fibrous cap becomes unstable, eventually allowing cholesterol and inflammatory cells to spill out into the lumen of the artery, either blocking blood flow (heart attack) or sending a clot downstream (stroke). Genetic susceptibility for heart disease is a problem. It is known there are about 100 abnormal genes which increase the risk for heart attacks and strokes. This accounts for only about 20% of the cases of cardiovascular disease. The other 80% is caused by lifestyle — things we do or are exposed making the vascular disease progress.

Vascular disease with cholesterol deposits in the coronary (heart) arteries and the aorta (the main blood vessel in the center of the body) have been found in young adults as early as 15 years of age. The standard American lifestyle creates a situation where endothelial dysfunction occurs early in life and progresses often unnoticed until the person has a heart attack or a stroke. A heart attack is indicated 62% of the time as the first sign of CVD (Cardiovascular Disease) in men and about 40% of the time in women. This is the reason many people who have been given a clean bill of health go on to develop a heart attack or stroke.

The traditional risk factors for CVD include high cholesterol, high blood pressure, diabetes, smoking, obesity, male gender, sedentary lifestyle and a positive family history of premature CVD. Often individuals may not have many of these traditional risk factors yet still end up with a heart attack or stroke. It is obvious that we are missing other risk factors that must be identified if we are going to help more people avoid CVD.

We know that a low anti-oxidant level in the blood is a risk factor. Antioxidants help decrease the damage caused by what are called reactive oxygen species (ROS). These are molecules that float around in the blood and cells that damage all parts of the cell including the mitochondria (which make energy) and the DNA (our genetic makeup). The best source of antioxidants is from a diet high in vegetables and fruits. The goal is to eat about six servings of vegetables per day and a few fruits. I recommend limiting the fruit since excess sugar in the body is converted and stored as fat.

Cholesterol is another risk factor; specifically, it is the LDL cholesterol (bad cholesterol) and more so when the LDL is oxidized. Anything that injures the LDL molecules causing oxidation (this is like rusting of the LDL particles) increases plaque formation in the arteries. When oxidized LDL gets into the wall of the arteries called the Intima, it stimulates an abnormal inflammatory reaction allowing plaque to build up.

131

While dyslipidemia is a risk factor including elevated total cholesterol, elevated triglycerides and oxidized LDL, the size and number of the LDL particles are probably more significant. Smaller LDL particles can easily get into the walls of the arteries creating inflammation, thickening, buildup of cholesterol and cellular debris and resultant damage.

HDL is known as the good cholesterol yet when it gets too high, it becomes dysfunctional meaning good cholesterol is less able to do its job of clearing LDL from the blood. Diabetes is a risk factor and as the fasting glucose increases above 75, the risk of CVD is also higher. Also, when the insulin level is high, it is another CVD risk factor.

High sugar in the diet stimulates a similar inflammatory reaction in the walls of the arteries. This is the reason individuals with diabetes have more heart attacks and strokes. Studies have shown that inflammation occurs after a meal (post prandial hyperglycemia/ elevated blood sugar) when the meal includes a lot of simple sugars (refined carbohydrates).

Vitamin deficiencies also represent another risk factor for CVD. One of the most important chemicals for normal arterial function is nitric oxide (NO). This chemical keeps arteries dilated, making it easy for blood to flow through them. B-complex vitamins are necessary for nitric oxide production; when a person is deficient in specific nutrients, CVD develops.

As stated above, high blood pressure is a traditional risk factor for heart disease. Often people are not aware of the significance of slight elevations in blood pressure, how they affect the endothelium, and the risk of heart disease and strokes. The risk starts at a blood pressure of about 110/70; research has shown that for every increase in systolic/diastolic BP of 20/10, there is a doubling of the risk for heart attack and stroke. An increase from 110/70 to 130/80 escalates the risk; and, it gets worse as the pressure increases. High blood pressure, therefore, is actually a marker for endothelial dysfunction. To decide on the proper treatment, we must understand and deal with the cause of the high blood pressure.

Visceral fat is another risk factor — the fat that accumulates around the internal organs. Fat cells create dozens of inflammatory chemicals which increase the risk not only of CVD, but also make the individual more susceptible to diabetes, hypertension and other metabolic diseases.

Stress, anxiety, depression and even sleep deprivation are other risk factors. These situations create hormone imbalance that leads to dysfunction of the endothelium. Obstructive sleep apnea is a condition where the individual stops breathing for short periods of time at night; this increases the risk for irregular heart rhythms and high blood pressure in the lungs.

Abnormal protein spilling into the urine (called micro albuminuria) is another marker of endothelial dysfunction. This indicates the blood vessels within the kidneys are injured, allowing protein to be lost into the urine. A simple blood test called C-reactive protein (CRP) is a sign of inflammation within the body; it can be used over time as a marker for improvement while we treat the inflammation. Excess alcohol and soda are other risk factors. A homocysteine blood test indicates the levels of B-complex vitamins which, as mentioned above, are a risk factor when deficient. When we look at nutrition as a risk factor, we know that diets high in saturated fat and trans fats are concerning. The hormone DHEA, when low, is a risk factor as is low testosterone or high estrogen in a male. Hormone risk factors in women include low estrogen and low progesterone.

Hypothyroidism is a CVD risk factor for both men and women. Low magnesium, low chromium and low iron in the blood are others. Even periodontal disease is a risk factor because of the abnormal bacteria which accumulates in the mouth and sets up a condition of systemic inflammation (inflammation throughout the body). It is important to realize that risk factors for heart disease are also risk factors for brain disease. Many of the same factors that positively and negatively affect the heart also affect the brain.

Recently I have written about low Vitamin K2 levels as a risk factor. This is because vitamin K2 helps move calcium into the bones; when the level of K2 is low, calcium moves into the arteries rather than the bones, making the arteries stiff and less compliant.

MPO/Myeloperoxidase and the PLAC test are other specific blood tests which give information about the amount of inflammation in and around the arterial wall and the vulnerability of the plaque, meaning how likely it is to rupture. These are advanced tests which clarify what is happening at the endothelial level. This is where heart disease starts. Since this is a long-term process, it is important to know when it begins, stop the progression and reverse the process quickly.

Low levels of Coenzyme Q10 are a CVD risk factor as this enzyme is necessary for the production of energy (ATP) in all cells, especially in the heart. Low vitamin D is a risk factor, not only for CVD but also for many brain/neurodegenerative diseases, cancer and other chronic illnesses. Vitamin D acts more like a hormone than a vitamin; and, is known to have hundreds of functions throughout the body.

The coronary calcium score (CCS) evaluates the amount of calcium building up in the arteries and is a moderately early marker for endothelial dysfunction.

The point of this article is to help the reader understand there are many more risk factors for endothelial dysfunction and CVD than just the traditional risk factors. Once an individual has quantified his/her risk factors, the plan is to put in place changes to decrease the risks. The usual recommendations include eating heart healthy foods and drinks, exercising regularly, lowering the stress level, getting enough sleep and not smoking. In addition, we must ensure we have adequate levels of antioxidants, balanced hormones, avoid toxins as much as possible and bolster the immune system. Supplements such as CoQ 10, resveratrol and curcumin have been shown to protect the heart and brain. Metformin is a prescription medication used primarily for treatment of diabetes. It also has protective effects in cardio-metabolic disease; research indicates it increases longevity. Statin medications have been shown to lower cholesterol, LDL levels and may help to decrease inflammation.

Specific blood tests can be done to measure the levels of all vitamins, minerals and antioxidants; and, if any of these are found to be deficient, supplements may be used while remembering that micronutrients should come primarily from what we eat. If we eat a clean diet and are still deficient in micronutrients, then taking supplements will round out the action plan.

As we age, all hormones except the stress hormone, cortisol, decrease, making it important to have our hormone levels checked. We know from clinical studies that hormone replacement (rebalancing) lowers the risk, not only cardiac and vascular problems, it also lowers the risk for neurodegenerative diseases and helps people live a longer and better-quality life.

In summary, the evaluation of individuals for early cardio-metabolic disease and endothelial dysfunction is possible analyzing traditional risk factors and many of the more comprehensive risk factors as detailed above. Once the health of the endothelium is known, the physician and the patient can develop a comprehensive action plan to improve overall health and longevity.

- Dr. Sal

Are Genetically Modified Foods (GMOs) Safe?

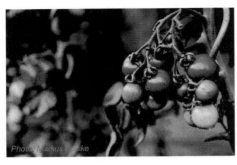

The National Academies of Science (NAS) recently reported on the safety of genetically modified foods (aka GE/ genetically engineered foods) stating that they are safe for human and animal consumption. Since there has been so much controversy on this topic, it is important to review the science.

Fifty experts from this non-profit group (NAS) took two years to review 900 studies done on GE foods from the past 20 years since GE crops were introduced. They listened to 80 people who had diverse expertise, experience and perspectives on genetically engineered (GE) crops to augment the diversity of those represented by this committee. These experts also reviewed 700 comments and documents from individuals and organizations about the risks and benefits of GE crops. In addition, the committee reviewed research reports regarding the same.

The group acknowledged that some members of the public are skeptical about the research that has been done since many of the experiments have been completed by industries that are profiting from these crops. The report is said to highlight the affiliations of the primary researchers and the specific sources of the funding. This information is available on the web site: http://nas-sites.org/GE-crops/.

According to the report, this study was funded by the New Venture fund, the Gordon and Betty Moore Foundation, the Burroughs Wellcome Fund, the USDA and the NAS. I personally looked at the site to review the funding sources. Chapters four through six list the funding sources. In chapter four alone there are 155 research reports that do not list the funding source. Of the reports that did list their funding source, several researchers were found to be funded by the following: Monsanto (16 studies), the USDA (32 studies), Bayer and Novartis (pharmaceutical companies) and others. Chapters five and six revealed similar results including companies such as Dow Chemical and DuPont.

There may be a link between agricultural, chemical and pharmaceutical companies that benefit from producing the GE seeds, the pesticides and herbicides used on these crops. This includes medications needed to treat cancer and chronic diseases when they do occur. The NAS group consensus was that GMO crops were not responsible for increasing the incidence of cancer, obesity, GI illness, kidney disease, autism or allergies. It appears that prospective, randomized controlled, double blind studies (the standard type of research design) have not been done in humans.

The American Medical Association Council on Science and Public Health stated that "bioengineered foods have been consumed for 20 years and during that time no overt consequences to human health have been reported" — again, where are safety studies in humans?

In reviewing the NAS report, page 156 offers a conclusion about the effects of GE crops on human health: the research that has been concluded in studies with animals and on chemical composition of GE foods reveals no differences that would implicate a higher risk to human health from eating GE foods. Long-term epidemiological studies have not directly addressed GE food consumption effects on humans. How can these conclusions be made?

It is interesting to read about the USDA (U.S. Department of Agriculture) which is now made up of 29 agencies with 100,000 employees in 4,500 locations across the country and abroad. It was initially developed by President Lincoln in 1862 as The People's Department. The Food, Nutrition and Consumer Services Department of the USDA has as its mission to work to end hunger and improve health in the United States. The Food Safety Department mission of the USDA is to ensure that the Nation's supply of food is safe, wholesome and properly labeled. With these mandates, many people wonder why the health of the population in the U.S. continues to decline; and, why there still is no mandate on labeling GE foods. Shouldn't the public be aware of which foods are genetically engineered so they can make their own decisions? How can individuals be responsible for their own health if they do not have adequate information?

My concern with this report is that it is incomplete. Many of the funding sources are missing and the motives questionable while prospective research has not been done with humans. How do we know these GE foods are truly safe for humans to consume?

We can do something beneficial despite the above. We can continue to purchase and eat only non-GMO or non-GE foods. When we purchase fruits and vegetables, we should be looking for the non-GMO label; and, if the product does not have this designation, simply do not buy it. We must ensure that we are eating healthy food since nutrition is the one thing that will lead us down the road to either good health or disease. You may want to watch the You Tube video called *Genetic Roulette*.

The other positive idea is to let our voices be heard. Let your public officials know your thoughts on this subject. Insist on mandatory labeling of all GE/GMO foods. Buy organic produce as often as you can, follow the **Dirty Dozen** list — which is a list of the vegetables and fruits most contaminated by pesticides and herbicides. Even if you do not look at the list, remember if the fruit or vegetable has a thin skin, then the pesticides and herbicides are deeply absorbed, therefore, posing a health risk. If it has a thin skin, buy organic! It is worth the extra money. As I tell everyone, you will either pay now for healthy food or you will pay later for medicine, doctor visits, hospitalizations and even more devastating, in lost years of quality life. Shopping at the local farmers' markets cuts the expense significantly since most of the local growers produce organic crops.

Health care reform starts with each one of us. We are responsible for our own health and maintaining our health should be the number one priority every day. I can almost guarantee every person reading this article agrees it is much easier to avoid disease as opposed to treating disease once it has occurred. In most cases, treatment never gets the person back to optimal health. A cure for many diseases simply does not exist. It is true that traditional health care has come a long way in the last 100 years; yet, it is also true that most of the health problems we deal with today are the result of how we live and what we are exposed to. Better health, improved quality of life and greater longevity may be attained by not exposing ourselves to what many believe are the harmful effects of GE foods.

- Dr. Sal

The Pros and Cons of Dietary Protein

Protein is one of the essential macro nutrients in the same category as carbohydrates and fats. Macro nutrients are the building blocks for all the cells in the body. In addition to macro nutrients, the body also needs what are called micro nutrients which include all the vitamins and minerals that are required by the cells to use the proteins, fats and carbohydrates we eat. Proteins, fats and carbohydrates are used to make components of all cells and the micro nutrients are enzymes that allow these chemical reactions to happen.

Once the protein source passes from the mouth and esophagus into the stomach, hydrochloric acid (HCL) activates the enzyme, pepsin, which starts the process of converting protein into amino acids. The amino acids are then absorbed and transported throughout the body. Once taken up by cells, in addition to forming parts of the cells, amino acids are used to make hormones, brain enzymes and other chemicals essential for the normal function of the body and brain.

Proteins have many other varied functions: cell growth and repair, maintenance of hair, nails, muscles, bones, formation of enzymes, hormones and fluid balance. The production of antibodies is also an essential part of the immune system. Proteins act as a later source of energy. It is important to understand that we do not want the body to be using protein as an energy source; the body should use fat for energy production. When we begin to move around in the morning, the body utilizes glucose, an immediate source of energy.

Once inside the cells, the protein is metabolized using micro nutrients (vitamins and minerals). This process also requires growth hormone (GH). This is a hormone produced mainly at night while we

140

sleep. GH helps the body use the proteins we eat to improve the health of skeletal muscles, bones and all the cells in our body.

As mentioned, protein digestion requires HCL, which is produced in the stomach. Many people use proton pump inhibitors (PPIs) such as Prilosec to lower acid production in their stomach to the point where digestion and absorption of amino acids is hampered. I usually counsel my patients to find the cause of their heartburn; we often find that it comes from taking in too many unhealthy food and drink products. The treatment for heartburn/reflux is to remove the offending agent such as spicy foods, too much alcohol, coffee and sweets. Once this is done, the medication may not be needed, and the side effects of these medications are alleviated. The TV commercials for PPI medications do not highlight the fact that they can cause osteoporosis, an increased risk for pneumonia and leaky gut syndrome — remove the cause of the heartburn and all is well!

Dietary protein sources include all animal meats, dairy, vegetables, nuts and seeds. Protein powders are made from whey (cow's milk) protein as well as vegetable sources. Many people do not realize that on a calorie-per-calorie basis, there is more protein in vegetables compared to beef, chicken or pork. This is because the meat products also contain fat which actually make up more of the calories than the protein. Whey protein is cow's milk protein and the concern I have with this source of protein is the relationship to osteoporosis. According to the research, whey protein makes the blood more acidic and increases the risk for bone breakdown (osteoporosis).

According to many of the national organizations the protein requirement is 0.8 - 1.5 grams per kilogram which means that a male weighing 150 lbs. (70 kg) would require 56-105 grams per day. The higher amounts would be for a person doing moderately intense exercise on a regular basis. If a person is doing extreme exercise, then the total amount needed increases beyond 105 grams.

Protein digestion, absorption and utilization are finely tuned processes that require many different moving parts. It is important to understand the intricacies of this process and why eating and drinking healthy proteins, while also getting the proper number of various vitamins and minerals, is vital for optimal health.

We must be aware of the ramifications of eating or drinking too much protein. The body takes the protein required to repair cell damage, make new cells, produce hormones and chemicals as mentioned and it essentially stores protein as skeletal muscle. If the intake exceeds the needs of the body, the protein has to be removed in a healthy way. The kidneys are the organs that deal with this excess and when the levels of protein in the body get too high, the kidneys begin to fail. The medical term is renal insufficiency; as the condition progresses, we use the term renal/kidney failure.

Recently I read an article about a Strongman Competition where one of the competitors had a diet which included several hundred grams of protein per day. Like many other situations in which a person abuses his or her body, this can be tolerated for a short time. In the long term, however, this amount of protein will damage a person's kidneys, placing the person at risk for renal insufficiency and even renal failure.

In summary, the take-home message is: we all need protein. Protein is essential for life — we need a certain amount, yet not too much. Vegetables provide more protein calorie for calorie. If you prefer to get your protein from animal sources, be sure it is antibiotic free, grass fed and not contaminated with pesticides, herbicides or fecal bacteria which is very common, especially in chicken meat. If you eat a lot of soy protein, make sure it is not genetically modified (non-GMO). Limit protein intake depending on the amount and intensity of exercise you do and visit with your primary care physician regularly for a blood test that checks the function of your kidneys. It is important to get 7-8 hours of quality sleep nightly to make enough growth hormone allowing you to use the protein to keep your body and brain strong and functional.

- Dr. Sal

Neurodegenerative Diseases

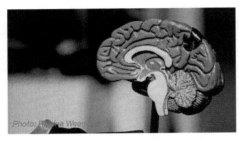

Photo: _____

We can learn about neurodegenerative (brain) diseases, about the etiology, the signs, symptoms, treatment; yet, even more important is the prevention. Let's start with the most common neurodegenerative disease (NDD) that Muhammad Ali suffered from, namely Parkinson's disease (PD). Next is one of the most common NDDs, Alzheimer's dementia. Other NDDs include multi-infarct/vascular dementia, multiple sclerosis, as well as traumatic brain injury.

Parkinson's disease (PD) is a movement disorder. It is caused by decreased production of dopamine from an area of the brain called the *substantia nigra*. Deficiency in dopamine results in the following problems: moving the upper and lower extremities, a slowness of movement and sometimes freezing where the person is unable to move for a short period, weakness of the muscles controlling facial expression, weakness swallowing, tremors which may involve the hands or the head, problems with handwriting, sleeping and constipation. There are medications for PD, but the effect is less than complete and may slow the progression — a cure is less likely.

Alzheimer's dementia (AD) is the most common type of dementia in older adults. AD causes problems with cognition – thinking, reasoning and remembering. It also causes behavioral problems and as brain function declines, AD results in significant problems for the person to maintain normal activities of daily living. There is a genetic component to AD in a minority of cases. The etiology (cause) is unknown but appears to be related to other metabolic diseases such as cardiovascular disease, strokes, hypertension, diabetes and even obesity. Similar to PD, there are medications for AD that are less than effective; therefore, the emphasis has to be on preventing the disease.

Multi-infarct/vascular dementia is caused by multiple small infarcts (mini strokes) in the brain. Vascular dementia indicates the brain is not getting the proper amount of blood flow; this can be the result of many small strokes occurring over time or the development of arteriosclerosis (hardening of the arteries) in the vessels of the brain. The person with multi-infarct dementia (MID) develops problems with brain function over a period of years. This occurs slowly while the person and the family might not even notice what is happening. The decline in brain function is often attributed to aging yet this is not a normal part of aging. In many cases, similar to AD, MID is related to the person also having cardiovascular disease (CVD) or diabetes. These are diseases that clog the arteries, not allowing normal blood flow to the brain. The treatment for MID is similar to the treatment for CVD – controlling the cholesterol and blood pressure, eating whole foods and getting regular exercise. It is important to focus on a healthy lifestyle since the etiology of MID is more related to lifestyle behaviors than genetics.

MID may be related to hypertension (high blood pressure). This is especially problematic since high blood pressure in most cases is asymptomatic, meaning no symptoms. High blood pressure in the brain can be associated with aneurysms in the arteries of the brain. An aneurysm is a small out-pouching of an artery similar to what happens to a balloon when a small area of the balloon weakens and pops out. When the blood pressure is high, the aneurysm can burst releasing blood into the brain, causing a buildup of pressure which then affects normal brain function. Since the brain is held in a small confined cavity (the skull), it cannot tolerate any significant increases in pressure before it becomes severely affected. Hemorrhage of blood into the brain is an emergency and can be fatal, if not treated immediately. This situation represents a brain attack; when this occurs, 911 should be the first call since there are many things a neurosurgeon can do to help.

Multiple sclerosis is one of the most devastating neurologic disorders in young people. It occurs as a result of demyelination of various areas in the brain and spinal cord. Myelin is the covering of nerve cells and when myelin is lost, the nerves cannot function normally. The demyelination comes and goes in various regions of the brain and this causes different symptoms such as numbness, weakness and coordination problems. There are four distinct types of MS related to the progression. Some people develop a relapsing and remitting course, others develop a more progressive course. Other symptoms include fatigue, tingling, weakness, dizziness, vertigo, pain and bladder weakness with urinary tract infections. Again, as with many of the other neurodegenerative diseases, treatment is limited, less than optimal and certainly not curative.

Traumatic brain injury (TBI) is another neurodegenerative disease which is caused by either a single acute injury to the brain or from repeated, apparently smaller insults. When a person develops an acute injury to the brain, they may develop a concussion (a bruise on the brain) which in some cases resolves completely yet prolonged or even permanent damage may occur. When a child playing football or soccer gets a head concussion, we know that with each successive concussion, the risk of permanent damage increases. There have been many cases recently in the news of professional football players developing AD after years of playing football and having multiple concussions. This appears to be part of the problem that occurred with Mohammed Ali. Although he was diagnosed with PD, many people believe a majority of his brain problems were related to multiple head injuries and concussions. It only makes sense that continued pounding to the head will eventually result in permanent degeneration of brain function. Many more cases of TBI occur because of motor vehicle and other accidents, falls and violence. This is a very common problem in young individuals resulting in cognitive, social, emotional and behavioral problems, which can be temporary or permanent.

Having looked at the most common types of neurodegenerative diseases, we realize the treatment of these disorders is not encouraging. Prevention is the key to all health problems; it is much easier to prevent illnesses as opposed to attempting to treat or cure them. With brain illness we can prevent problems by doing the following: first, do not injure the brain. For those who ride motorcycles, WEAR A HELMET! Your brain cannot tolerate much damage, so protect it! Next, consider not playing sports that result in repeated head injuries. It is not worth any amount of fun that can be had by participating in a sport that can ruin your life as an adult. Limiting exposure to toxins also helps; these include alcohol, recreational drugs and heavy metals such as mercury which we are exposed to when we eat a lot of fish. Even some prescription medications over time can result in an increased risk.

On the positive side, we know that exercise helps the brain, as does eating whole foods. When we exercise regularly, we supply the brain with more blood, nutrients and oxygen. Eating whole foods gives the brain more nutrients and less toxins such as pesticides and herbicides. Limiting processed foods decreases the inflammation in the brain that occurs from all the chemicals in processed foods. The body and brain are not meant to deal with synthetic chemicals therefore, limiting the exposure is one of the best ways to prevent NDD. Sleep and stress management are also important. Quality sleep (7-8 hours per night) allows for the production of melatonin, an important hormone for health and longevity. Limiting stress decreases cortisol levels. When cortisol is chronically elevated, it affects the memory center in the brain (the hippocampus) leading to decreased memory and other chronic brain problems.

In summary, protecting the brain by living a healthy life is the best way to prevent neurodegenerative diseases and even when these problems do occur, research has shown that living a healthy life also helps with the treatment and the reversal of disease.

- Dr. Sal

Immune System Diseases

Over the past 100 years we have seen improvements and even eradication of some diseases such as small pox. We have also seen the rise of many other diseases and autoimmune diseases. It is estimated that there are about 100 different autoimmune diseases. By definition, these are diseases in which the body actually attacks itself. The normal response to infections or toxins is for the immune system to make antibodies which fight off the infection or to somehow metabolize the toxin. The body usually does this with efficiency; yet, sometimes the immune reaction goes awry and these antibodies end up injuring one's own tissues. These are examples of immune system over activity. The opposite may also occur; diseases occur when the immune system is functioning at a low level and unable to fully deal with infections, toxins or other insults. These are called immune-deficiency syndromes. With this explanation, we see that both spectrums of immune dysfunction may occur resulting in an array of different, life altering and sometimes fatal illnesses.

In this article we will review the diseases pertaining to over activity of the immune system. The normal immune response to something which triggers the immune system such as an infection, exposure to a toxin, is to produce antibodies. When dealing with a disease of immune over activity, instead of fighting an infection or getting rid of the toxin, these antibodies attack the host cells, i.e., the person's own cells. One concerning category of triggers is environmental chemicals. In reviewing the literature, I found that over the past century about 30,000 new chemicals have been produced and introduced into the environment. While it is not certain how accurate this number is, the reader can get a sense of the large number of chemicals simply by reading labels. If you start out at the grocery store and read labels on food products, you will be struck by the number of chemicals in foods. These chemicals are added as preservatives, food colorings, stabilizers and flavorings. These chemicals are ingested, absorbed across the gut wall into the blood stream; therefore, all the cells in the body are exposed. It is no wonder we see so many autoimmune diseases.

Some examples of common autoimmune disorders include: rheumatoid arthritis (RA), systemic lupus erythromatosis (SLE), Inflammatory bowel diseases such as ulcerative colitis (UC) and Crohn's disease, Type 1 diabetes, Graves' disease (thyroid) as well as Hashimoto's thyroiditis, multiple sclerosis (MS), psoriasis, myasthenia gravis and different types of vasculitis.

Rheumatoid arthritis (RA) occurs when the immune system produces antibodies which attack the lining of the joints causing inflammation, pain, swelling and joint destruction. If untreated, RA causes permanent joint damage and disability.

Lupus (SLE) is a condition where the body produces antibodies that attack the lungs, kidneys, blood vessels and nerves. Since this is a systemic disease, it causes widespread organ and tissue injury; in some cases, may cause life threatening organ damage.

Inflammatory bowel diseases such as ulcerative colitis and Crohn's disease are common autoimmune diseases of the GI tract. These diseases cause significant problems with bloody bowel movements, diarrhea, malabsorption, abdominal pain, anemia, unintentional weight loss, as well as an increased risk for colon cancer.

Type 1 diabetes occurs when antibodies attack the pancreas, an organ which is just behind the stomach and responsible for making insulin. When the body does not make the necessary amount of insulin, blood glucose levels rise, and the person suffers from many different problems which may lead to blindness, kidney failure, amputations, heart attacks and early death.

Graves' disease occurs when antibodies attack the thyroid gland causing it to release excess thyroid hormone, leading to hyperthyroidism. The individual might experience unintentional weight loss, a rapid heart rate, irritability, weakness, brittleness of the hair and nails.

Hashimoto's thyroiditis sounds similar to Graves; but, as the antibodies attack the thyroid gland, the initial effect is hyperthyroidism (rapid excess thyroid hormone release) which is then followed by a hypothyroid (low thyroid) state as the gland is no longer able to release hormones. The end result is chronic fatigue, weight gain, constipation, dry skin, sensitivity to cold; and, if the hypothyroid state is untreated, it may even result in congestive heart failure.

Multiple sclerosis is an immune condition where antibodies attack nerve cells in the brain and spinal cord. The symptoms dictate which nerve cells are involved. A person might have numbness in the fingers at one time and then another time have problems with vision or moving a limb. The signs and symptoms are fleeting – they come and go. In some cases, the condition is progressive while in other cases, symptoms occur and then resolve without permanent damage. Stress, heat and possibly infections may reoccur.

Psoriasis is an over-active condition involving T-cells (specialized immune cells). When the T-cells are over activated, damage occurs in the skin, giving it a silvery appearance with plaques (thickening of the skin) which form over the elbows, backs of the knees and over the lower part of the scalp.

Myasthenia gravis (MG) is another autoimmune condition which affects the nerves leading to generalized weakness of the skeletal muscles. The hallmark is muscle weakness that increases during periods of activity and decreases when at rest. Muscles controlling facial expression, chewing and swallowing as well as control of eyelid function and eye movements often occur. Muscles that control head and limb movement and breathing can be affected.

Vasculitis is an inflammation of the blood vessels and another example of an autoimmune disease. Inflammation causes problems with blood flow because of thickening and scarring. Symptoms occur as blood flow to various organs and tissues is decreased. When the cells of the body are not supplied with the proper amount of oxygen and nutrients, they become injured and over time the cells die. Entire organs may fail and if this involves multiple areas of the body, this type of autoimmune disease may be fatal.

Temporal arteritis is an example of a vasculitis which affects the temporal arteries that are located along the side of the head lateral to the corner of the eye. The temporal artery supplies the eye with blood; when inflammation occurs, the person is at risk for blindness.

Regardless of the specific autoimmune disease, the treatment is usually some type of medication which suppresses the over-active immune response. With these treatments, care must be taken to make sure the person does not become immunosuppressed, meaning that the immune function is so low that the person is less able to respond normally to infections. This is one of the biggest concerns when using these types of prescription medications. It becomes a balancing act to ensure the person gets the proper amount of suppression, yet not too much. Close contact with the physician prescribing these medications is essential. The individual is usually instructed to call his/her physician with any signs or symptoms of infection such as fever, chills and sweats. The goal is to suppress the abnormal immune reaction without impairing the normal immune function.

When dealing with a health problem, always look for the cause of the problem; then look to see if there is a lifestyle behavior which may be used to treat the cause. It is most important to look for triggers of an autoimmune reaction. It might be exposure to the following: chemicals in food, pesticides on fruits and vegetables, contaminants in the water we drink or from chemicals leaching from the plastic water bottles, herbicides used on shrubs and lawn, chemicals in cosmetics, over-the-counter as well as prescription medications, recreational drugs and tobacco. If you detoxify, you may be able to prevent an autoimmune reaction in the first place. If you already have an autoimmune reaction, by living a clean life, you may be able to more effectively treat and possibly reverse an existing autoimmune disease.

- Dr. Sal

What Are Common Reasons For Chronic Fatigue?

Many people seem to complain of a lack of energy; they describe the feeling of always being tired. Most of the time people just ignore this and keep going, assuming that fatigue is due to the 24/7/365 lifestyle that we lead in the U.S. Frequently, this might be due to an underlying health problem which should be diagnosed and properly treated.

It is important to understand there are many medical problems which may lead to chronic fatigue. That is why we encourage you to see your physician/health care provider if you are suffering from chronic fatigue.

Low thyroid is one of the most common reasons many people believe to be the cause of their tiredness. Certainly, this is part of the differential diagnosis for chronic fatigue. When being considered, this is diagnosed with a simple blood test. There are actually several tests run as part of the thyroid panel, including the levels of T4 (the pro-hormone), T3 (the active hormone) and TSH, the regulator hormone released from the brain; this is sent to the thyroid gland to control the production and release of thyroid hormone. When thyroid hormone levels are decreased, the person feels tired, might gain weight, hair and nail strength start to diminish. If this is not corrected, heart function may decline, making the person more susceptible to heart failure.

Low testosterone is another reason for chronic fatigue. Testosterone is the male hormone for sexual development and function. It is important to understand that females also need a certain amount of testosterone to age in a healthy way. When the testosterone level is low, the individual lacks a sense of wellbeing, muscle and bone strength declines, mood changes can occur and the risk of depression

154

increases. Checking the level of free/active testosterone is another blood test; replacement with bio-identical testosterone works well to get the level back into a healthy range. The goal in replacing hormones is to get the level up to an optimal range where maximal function can occur. The goal is to optimize health and not just to prevent disease.

Sleep deprivation is another obvious cause of chronic fatigue; not only limited hours of sleep, but also decreased quality of sleep. As many people get older, they frequently get up at night to urinate. Frequent interruptions in sleep decrease the quality of the sleep, making it difficult to feel rested in the morning. This also interferes with the production of growth hormone which is made at night and necessary for the maintenance of healthy muscles, bones and weight.

Depression is an under-diagnosed cause of chronic fatigue. Often an individual hesitates to talk with their physician about depression or may not even realize symptoms of depression. When the physician starts to evaluate a person complaining of chronic fatigue, they look for the common illnesses; in this evaluation, depression is also considered a cause, especially if the work up for physical illness is non-revealing. If it is apparent that depression might be the reason for the chronic fatigue, the initial part of the treatment is to identify the reason for the depression. It might be due to a recent traumatic life event, a bad relationship or loss of a job, to name a few. Once the reason for the depression is identified, then psychological counseling is often helpful. Sometimes antidepressant medications can be helpful; yet, if they simply mask the cause of the problem (treating only the symptom), they could make the fatigue worse.

Iron and/or B12 deficiency are other common reasons for chronic fatigue. Many times, females develop iron deficiency anemia secondary to heavy menstrual periods. B12 deficiency is usually due to poor nutrition. Replacement of iron and B12 to correct the anemia is then necessary. In some situations, a person with iron deficiency

155

anemia requires consultation with a gastrointestinal specialist who looks for blood loss in the GI tract.

Stress is another common cause of chronic fatigue which may be a result of low cortisol. When stress is persistent, the adrenal glands continually produce and release the cortisol hormone. Over time the adrenal glands begin to fail, resulting in what is called adrenal fatigue. Diagnosis of this problem requires either a 24-hour urine collection or several blood tests done over a 24-hour period. Similar to the plan for depression, finding the cause of the stress and working to eliminate it usually helps eliminate the adrenal dysfunction and the chronic fatigue.

There are many prescription medications which can cause fatigue including beta blockers (used for heart problems and high blood pressure), anti-depressants as mentioned above, anti-anxiety medications, attention deficit disorder medications, etc. Keeping a diary of symptoms is often helpful in determining if a newly started medication is causing side effects. If there seems to be a relationship between starting a medication and the development of symptoms (i.e., chronic fatigue), speak with your physician before making any adjustments.

Poor nutrition is a very common reason for a lack of energy. Think of the nutrition in food as fuel for your gas tank. If you put the lowest grade of gasoline in your car, then the engine will not work at maximum efficiency. The same is true for the body (your engine). When you eat low quality foods (processed, high in salt, sugar and fat), the mitochondria (parts of the cells where energy is made) do not function normally and cannot make enough energy to maintain all the vital functions of the body and brain. Overall function suffers and the individual complains of always being tired. This is one of the reasons I recommend eating six servings of organic vegetables daily that are filled with the essential vitamins, minerals, antioxidants, proteins, fats, carbohydrates and fiber we need to stay healthy.

Lack of exercise is another reason for chronic fatigue. The more a person does not exercise, the more they become de-conditioned and have less energy. The general recommendation is doing at least 30 minutes of moderately intense exercise daily, including aerobic and weight lifting/resistance exercises. Before starting an exercise program, it is important to consult with your physician to be sure you are healthy enough. Many adults require a stress test before starting exercise to ensure they do not have any underlying heart disease. Once this is done, starting slowly and advancing the exercise program under the supervision of an exercise specialist is helpful.

It should be clear that there are many reasons for chronic fatigue. The recommendation is to visit your physician/health care provider if low energy is a chronic problem. The reason for the chronic fatigue   becomes apparent after a comprehensive history, physical examination, blood and other tests are performed. Once a diagnosis is made and a treatment plan is determined, the energy starts to return getting the individual back to maximal function again!

- Dr. Sal

Hormones Matter for Weight Management

Many Americans are dealing with a weight crisis; one of the concerning facts is that more young adults, adolescents and even younger children are becoming obese. We are now seeing younger people with type 2 diabetes which until recently has been a disease of older adults. The reason for this epidemic is the poor quality of food many people eat and in addition to the number of calories of food eaten, we have to look at the effects that particular foods have on the hormones that control metabolism and weight.

The hormones which influence body weight include leptin and ghrelin. This process also includes insulin, growth hormone, testosterone, DHEA and others. When working as it has been designed, the hormone system is a symphony. When they are in balance, they work in concert — the music is beautiful!

Ghrelin is the hormone that makes us hungry and leptin is released when the body has enough calories/fuel. It tells the brain we are full and slows the appetite. Insulin is one of the hormones which controls the glucose (sugar) level in the blood and is also indirectly involved in the formation and storage of fat. Growth hormone and testosterone are involved in the growth of healthy skeletal muscles. Since this is where we burn a lot of calories, it is important to have more muscle on your bones (skeleton) than fat. This is the reason weight lifting is recommended as part of a healthy exercise routine. The more muscles you have (and the less fat), the more efficient your body is burning calories.

Proteins, fats and carbohydrates are classified as macronutrients which are the building blocks for the body; they have different effects on the hormones which control metabolism and

158

weight. High quality protein has a beneficial effect on the hormone glucagon (which helps stabilize blood glucose/sugar) and the neurotransmitter dopamine (the brain chemical which makes us feel well). This is in contrast to carbohydrates which affect the hormone insulin. When we eat too many carbohydrates, especially high glycemic carbs, the level of insulin increases rapidly, causing a rapid transfer of glucose into the muscles and liver. In the muscles, glucose is used as energy yet, once the body uses what it needs for energy, the excess sugar is stored as fat. In the liver, the excess glucose is converted into triglycerides which also becomes stored as fat. Foods high in fiber will slow absorption of glucose and are beneficial for metabolism and weight control.

A good rule to follow is to have 30% protein and about 40% of low glycemic (slowly absorbed) carbohydrates with the remainder from high quality fats. Protein sources include lean meats, quinoa, nuts and seeds, protein powders as well as vegetables. Yes, vegetables contain protein. If you compare calorie for calorie, vegetables actually have more protein than meat; all meats are primarily fat and not just protein. If we look at the overall nutritional quality of meat protein — including chicken — considering all the contaminants such as pesticides, antibiotics and bacteria — meat protein is a lower quality protein compared to organic vegetables, nuts, seeds and soy/tofu proteins.

The glycemic index indicates how rapidly a food product increases the blood glucose. After a food product is digested and absorbed from the GI tract into the blood stream, the level of glucose increases; this stimulates the release of insulin from the pancreas. If the level of glucose increases rapidly, the pancreas has to quickly release more insulin to keep the level of glucose in a healthy range. This rapid increase in blood glucose and insulin is then followed by a rapid lowering of glucose. This is when the person starts to develop hunger cravings again. This becomes a cycle, resulting in storage of calories and weight gain. There are many online lists of low glycemic carbohydrates which are healthier since they are slowly digested and absorbed causing fewer fluctuations in blood glucose and insulin, resulting in less effect on weight and metabolism.

Once we are sure about eating healthier proteins and the right amount of carbs, what about the fats? Many people focus on lowering the fat content in their meals yet, sometimes this may be detrimental. We need a certain amount of fat in the diet since the nervous system and the hormonal system rely on fats to make cell linings, produce hormones, support the immune system and for overall general health. From a hormone perspective, if you do not intake enough healthy fats and cholesterol, the body may become deficient in the various hormones essential for optimal health. All hormone production requires cholesterol. If the level is too low, it is harder for the body to make estrogen, testosterone, DHEA, cortisol and other essential hormones.

The key is eating healthy fats such as avocado, nuts, seeds, olives, salmon and anchovies. Healthy fats feed the brain and the nervous system as well as support the endocrine/hormone and immune system. Research shows that hormone deficiencies increase the risk and incidence of all chronic diseases, cancers and shorten lives. When hormones are balanced, the individual lives longer and lives a better-quality life with less illness and risk of cancer.

Many readers have heard the saying *a calorie is a calorie* — when it comes to weight control and staying healthy, this statement is just plain false! Consider the consequences of eating 2000 calories per day of McDonald's food versus eating 2000 calories of fresh vegetables, some fruits, whole grain bread, fish, and nuts. Which meal do you think would make you feel more energetic and healthier? The goal is to take in highly nutritious food that is low in calories. By definition this includes all-natural foods as detailed above. When processed foods are avoided, the body is then supplied with high octane fuel that allows the engine to run at maximum efficiency.

In relation to how calories affect the hormone system, we check the blood levels of the hormones involved with nutrition and then balance them by eating healthy food as well as exercise, sleep and stress management. Testing for hormonal balance can be done with a simple blood test yet, to get a comprehensive assessment, often testing is done by checking the hormone levels in the saliva and urine. When hormone levels are checked by these three methods, the physician gets a complete look at the active hormones and how they are metabolized in the body. The goal is to have optimal levels of all hormones and ensure that the body is metabolizing (breaking down) these hormones into healthy chemicals able to be used to maintain optimal health. I use the word optimal to emphasize that health is not just about avoiding disease; it is about being as functional as possible at any age.

Optimal hormone balance requires a lifestyle action plan — focusing each day living healthy. Being aware of the foods eaten and asking yourself: will this food make me healthier or increase my risk for illness or cancer? Focus on adding 30 minutes of exercise into the daily routine, setting a time to go to sleep and to get out of bed in the morning, having a purpose in life and also managing stress. It means being grateful for all you have realizing there are always those less fortunate.

Life is about balance. When we live in such a way that the hormones in the body are balanced, we live better and longer. The calories we consume do make a difference and influence the hormonal balance of the body. Take care of your hormone system by living well — it will take care of you!

- Dr. Sal

Grow Up Without Getting Old!

Reading Between The Lines

While reading an edition of the *New York Times,* I came across several articles having to do with health, yet all were very different. The first was an article about the ability to sharply cut cancer risk by making small changes in lifestyle. The first paragraph was confusing since it stated, "unlike other things that kill us (cancer) seems to come out of nowhere." This is confusing since we know cancer risk increases with many things we come in contact with including: radiation, certain chemicals, tobacco, infections, even hormone changes. Knowing the factors that increase our risk for cancer certainly is important, since this allows us to modify our exposures and hopefully lower our risk for cancer. The article did explain the far majority of cancers appear not to be related to bad luck, rather to exposures which we have control over. The article ended with the suggestion that as we talk about cancer research, which will most likely cost billions of dollars and might not achieve the intended results, it is worth considering that in many cases prevention is not only the cheaper course, but also the most effective. Four domains were identified that are often noted to be related to disease prevention: smoking, exercise, obesity, and alcohol. Since these are all controllable risk factors, we must keep this in mind when developing a lifestyle which decreases the risk of cancer.

What we eat influences the risk for cancer and many other chronic illnesses. In this same edition of the *Times,* there was an article on the flawed food labeling bill explaining that the Senate was expected to vote on a bill requiring businesses to label genetically modified foods. This bill would allow companies to use electronic codes for scanning instead of simply labeling the foods as non-GMO.

Consumers would have to scan a barcode with their smart phone or scanners in the store to find out if the food product they are considering is genetically modified. The bill would require these labels on genetically modified soybeans and refined oils, but not all GMOs. The author of this article went on to write, "exempting large categories of genetically modified foods would make the labels useless." I recently wrote an article about GMOs and certainly agree with this last statement. How are we to make intelligent decisions about the foods we purchase and eat if we do not have correct information? Nutrition is the foundation of healthy living. We know that unhealthy food results in more cancer and chronic illness; and conversely, healthy eating leads to less disease — a longer and better-quality life. Prescription drugs are not always the answer to health problems, while healthy food is.

A third article in the paper, *Consumer and Drug Share Nudge the Market Higher*, explained what has been happening with pharmaceutical stocks. The stocks are certainly good for investors yet, is this really good for the health of the country? I believe the answer is two-fold. First, we must always give thanks to the scientists and clinical researchers who continually develop medications which treat, reverse and cure many illnesses. Health care in the past 100 years has progressed immensely due in large part to the development of blockbuster medications. With this has come a reliance on medications as a cure-all. A while ago, I wrote an article about gastric reflux. If you listen to TV commercials about this health problem (heartburn), all you need to do is take a pill and it will relieve the symptoms. Unfortunately, the commercial fails to recommend a change in eating as the cure! We can increase our retirement accounts by investing in pharmaceutical stocks, yet it is much better to invest in our health by living a healthy lifestyle. What is the sense of having a big nest egg when you retire, if you have poor health? My father ended the last years of his life suffering and dying from complications of many years of smoking. He was a great saver and investor, but he did not invest much into his health.

The last article was about a company that developed a blood test for detecting a gene mutation associated with a poor response to two drugs for the treatment of prostate cancer. This article was certainly appealing since being able to detect a person's capacity to respond to an anti-cancer drug is tremendous! This type of research allows for specific targeting of cancer cells and allows the oncologist (cancer specialist) to more effectively choose a medication that will treat an individual's cancer.

Health care has come a long way in the last 100 years. When we look at the advances in pharmaceuticals, procedures and surgeries, we have much to be thankful for. We have a long way to go in helping many lay people and health care providers alike to understand the value of living a healthy lifestyle. Part of the work being done by the members of the American College of Lifestyle Medicine (ACLM) is to develop criteria for physicians interested in using lifestyle medicine as part of the treatment and prevention strategies for their patients. This is the foundation for health. There are thousands of clinical research reports to support it. People live longer and more productive lives when they eat healthy food, exercise regularly, manage stress and get enough sleep. There are many other things we can do to maintain good health; that is what a lifestyle medicine physician/health care provider recommends to their patients.

- Dr. Sal

A Prescription for Change

My thanks go out to Dr. Neal Barnard, President of the Physicians Committee for Responsible Medicine, for continuing to teach physicians, health care providers and the general community about the importance of nutrition. In a recent edition of his journal, *Good Medicine*, Dr. Barnard highlights the clinical research evidence supporting the relationship between what we eat and our health. He reviews the science of nutrition leaving out his bias and his preferences. I applaud this approach and have been doing the same in my medical practice, my public presentations and in the articles I write. It is important for readers to understand Dr. Barnard and I are not trying to convince people to eat foods we prefer. The readers must make personal choices based on the scientific evidence. Dr. Barnard calls this a prescription for change; he emphasizes there is a sense of urgency since we are now living with an epidemic of diabetes, heart disease, obesity and many other chronic illnesses.

The incidence of these illnesses and others such as Alzheimer's and the dozens of autoimmune diseases continues to increase. We know that the large majority of these illnesses are related to nutrition and lifestyle considerably more than genetics. For all the chronic illnesses and many of the cancers, the 80:20 rule applies. This means that 80% of the time the cause is related to lifestyle behaviors (which are controllable) and only 20% to genetics. What is interesting about genetics is that our genes are not always our destiny! This means that even if you are born with genes that increase your susceptibility to an illness, you do not always have to develop the illness. Research has shown that a healthy lifestyle often is enough to keep these bad genes

165

turned off; therefore, some of the genetic susceptibility is also controllable – how exciting and empowering is this!

In the current edition of *Good Medicine*, Dr. Barnard writes,

> *"The United States research enterprise continues to favor pharmaceutical development, at the expense of critically needed studies addressing the nutritional causes of disease."*

I believe this is an accurate statement and whole-heartedly support it. Over the past six years I have delved into the science of nutrition and fully believe that the cause of most of the illnesses and many of the cancers many people suffer from today are the direct result of what they eat and how they live. I am sad to see this in my medical practice every day because many of the health problems my patients suffer from are preventable. These folks do not have to live with disease and disability; they are not aware of the tremendous impact food and lifestyle has on their health. During each office visit I spend a lot of time educating my patients on the value of healthy food, hopefully making them aware of the control they have on their own present and future health.

Dr. Barnard writes,

> *"Although many people are changing their diets and revolutionizing their health, many others still have no access to the information they need."*

This is where journals such as *Good Medicine* come in. The articles in this medical journal are written in such a way that even non-health care providers can understand and benefit from reading. I encourage the readers as well as physicians and other health care providers to read it since it reviews up-to-date research on the science of nutrition and the impact on our lives.

166

Dr. Kevin Hall has written an article in the journal, *Obesity*, regarding the impact of rapid weight loss on metabolism. The researchers in this study measured the metabolic rate of contestants on *The Biggest Loser* television weight loss program. They did this at the start, at the end of the challenge and again at a six-year follow up. They found a consistently slower metabolism as compared to before these folks started this weight- loss program. They all rapidly lost a lot of weight, their metabolic rates slowed, and some even had a decline in hormones which help control appetite.

What comes to mind after reading this study is the healthfulness of rapid weight loss. At least from this one study, it appears that rapid weight loss is not beneficial in the long run. Certainly, many will say this is the result of only one study -- yes, this is a valid point. I can relate to this since in my medical practice I now see mainly individuals attempting to lose a lot of weight. For many who lose a significant amount of weight in a short period, there are many who regain it quickly. The most effective is slow weight loss, about 1-2 lbs. per week combined with exercise, stress management and an intentional focus on maintaining a daily, healthy lifestyle. A comprehensive, healthy living action plan as the number one daily priority always wins out over a fad diet in the long term. Also, *The Biggest Loser* programs are not realistic. Many people who need to lose weight are unable to take months off to stay in a facility that makes them exercise many hours a day, feeds them only what they should eat and monitors their every action. This method of losing weight is neither realistic nor possible for most people; it does not teach anyone how to deal with their health problems while living in the real world. Our goal as health care providers is to teach people how to live a healthy life while they are living their lives, not escaping from them.

Dr. Barnard writes, we do need a *prescription for change*...a change in how we look at health problems, food, and make excuses for not exercising. Many rationalize, "I'm going to treat myself even though it's not the healthiest choice because I've worked hard all day and deserve it." In the U.S. today, many of us work a lot harder at our jobs than we do to stay healthy. After years of neglecting our health, we see it fail; many people say, "I guess I'm just getting old." When I hear this from some 50-year-old patients in my medical practice, I know we must change this mindset. At age 50, no one should think of themself as old. If this is the case, a person should take a hard look at their lifestyle and decide what needs to be changed to start feeling young again!

These individuals need a prescription for change. They need a prescription for healthy eating, a prescription for exercise and a prescription for a healthy lifestyle. Many Americans need an urgent prescription for change. It is important to understand that change happens. When we neglect our health, change comes in the form of disease, disability and early death. When we focus intentionally on making good health a priority, we take control over our lives. We prevent disease, stay young longer, live healthier and happier lives.

- Dr. Sal

Health Benefits of a Wellness Exam

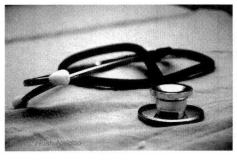

O ver the years there has been a debate about the benefits of a routine wellness examination. After practicing general Internal Medicine for over 25 years, I have no doubt this not only is beneficial, but necessary. Since the aging process affects individuals differently, we should all take advantage of a wellness physical examination. The blood, screening tests and diagnostic procedures available help the physician and health care providers understand the patient's health and future risks.

Health care and health problems have progressed over the past 50 years. Chronic illnesses and cancers continue to increase. In the past decades we have seen the development of over 100 autoimmune diseases. diseases. Cardiovascular diseases kill more people than any other illness, while cancers are close behind. In some countries, cancer has overtaken cardiovascular disease as the number one killer. Research has proven that most medical problems are more related to lifestyle than genetics yet, many people ignore the warnings and continue to live an unhealthy lifestyle.

What is interesting is that in the initial period when many people are living unhealthy lives, they believe they are healthy since they have not yet been diagnosed with a specific disease. They live believing they are healthy since they have no bad symptoms. They may be slowing down, but they attribute their slowing down to aging. Over time they develop shortness of breath with minimal activity and also attribute this to getting old. I have heard this from many people in their 40s and 50s and am truly amazed. This is just the beginning of middle age, not old age!

A wellness examination provides a significant benefit because it allows the physician the time to examine a person and, even more importantly, to identify health risk factors. In actuality, the wellness examination actually starts not with an examination, rather a conversation about how the individual is living. This gives the physician/health care provider clues to risk factors the individual has which will impact present and future health.

A typical patient might be a 50-year-old male working the customary 40-hour week and having no complaints. The physician then asks specific questions: "how's your energy, how many flights of stairs can you climb without getting short of breath, do you get any chest pains with activity, do you get any heartburn after eating?" The physician and the patient start to understand the person is not as healthy as he thinks. At 50 years of age, energy should not be a problem; climbing a few flights of stairs should not make a middle-aged man short of breath. Chest pain with activity is a sign of heart disease and not simply getting old. The heartburn after eating necessitates a change in dietary habits, possibly a gastroenterologist referral. After collecting this information, the physician begins to identify the possible reasons for these symptoms and early signs of disease. More questions are asked about lifestyle, specifically what the person eats on a regular basis, if he exercises and how often, his sleep pattern and how he deals with the normal stresses in life.

As a team, the physician and the patient talk about the use of tobacco, recreational drugs, prescription medications and other things that may influence the development of disease. When the actual physical examination begins, the physician might pick up a heart murmur, or hear what is called a carotid bruit indicating hardening of the carotid arteries that affects the supply of blood to the brain. Wheezing or decreased breath sounds when listening to the lungs of a smoker would indicate the need of a chest x-ray to rule out emphysema or lung cancer. When examining the abdomen of the patient, the physician may feel an enlarged liver, and on a blood test find very high cholesterol levels. If an excess of fat in the blood accumulates in the liver, it affects the function of the liver and may increase the person's risk for liver failure and cancer. The physician might recommend screening procedures such as a colonoscopy to rule out colon polyps or cancers, a mammogram for females and other tests to screen for hidden illnesses or even acute cancers. In the best case scenario, when no abnormalities are found, the physician may simply itemize the health risk factors and help develop an action plan to mitigate these risks.

This process enables the physician and patient to develop a relationship - one that will keep the person from developing illnesses and live a long healthy life. The goal of the physician is to help keep the patient healthy. It is the responsibility of the patient to do everything to stay well. One way is by getting a routine wellness examination.

My recommendation is for everyone over the age of 40 to have a wellness examination at least every other year, or annually if possible. In over 25 years as a physician I have had the honor of doing thousands of wellness exams and have found early disease in hundreds of people who thought they were healthy. Finding disease early allows us to intervene and make a real difference in the life of the person!

- Dr. Sal

Improving Health Through Sharing Great Information

A while ago I attended the International Conference on Nutrition in Medicine in Washington, DC, and listened to tremendously knowledgeable people talking about the potential of food to heal many of the health problems we deal with in America today.

Dr. Gerald Shulman spoke about the role of inflammation in diabetes and explained how fat accumulation within muscle cells contributes to insulin resistance, the precursor of diabetes. Also, fat accumulation in the liver of a person with uncontrolled diabetes is the leading cause of liver disease, resulting in a higher risk for cirrhosis and liver cancer. He explained that a weight loss of only 10% results in significant loss of fat from the liver and muscles, causing an improvement in liver and muscle function.

Dr. Kitt Peterson added to the discussion of insulin resistance and explained how this starts when a person gains weight and how insulin resistance is a significant risk factor for the number one killer in the U.S., namely cardiovascular disease. She explained how exercise improves insulin resistance; and, how this lowers the individual's risk for diabetes, heart disease and even dementia.

Dr. Stephen O'Keefe from the University of Pittsburgh spoke about the effects of nutrition on the GI system. He asked if a person could change their risk for colon cancer by changing what they eat — the answer is a resounding YES! He further explained the clinical research evidence linking colon cancer to red meat and processed meats (hot dogs, deli meats, sausage and bacon). He suggested (as did the recent report from the World Health Organization, or 'WHO') limiting these items in the diet, getting more fiber (which lowers the risk of colon cancer) and eating more vegetables and fruits.

172

Mariana Stern from the University of Southern California expanded on the WHO report and explained in detail where this information came from as well as the types of studies used to gather the information. The WHO study was a comprehensive, systematic review of the clinical data on cancer research and reached the conclusions as described in the previous paragraph. For more information on this extremely important topic, I refer the reader to the EPIC study and the AARP study which are the largest clinical studies regarding the association of nutrition and cancer.

The title of Christina Warinner's talk was Debunking the Paleo Myth. This was another exciting talk to listen to since so many people now are intrigued with the Paleo diet. She explained that humans have not evolved as carnivores and she discussed the anatomy of our teeth as compared to lions and other truly carnivorous animals. She also discussed the differences in our GI tracts, both anatomically and physiologically, and the differences in the types of digestive enzymes humans have as compared to carnivorous animals.

Meghan Jardine, from the Physicians Committee for Responsible Medicine, spoke next about the microbiome and diabetes. The microbiome is the bacterial environment within the GI tract that does many things to keep us healthy. She explained how the microbiome is injured by the use of antibiotics, when we eat processed foods and by using heartburn medications. When this occurs, the risk of diabetes, stomach cancers and other illnesses increase significantly. She explained healthy nutrition not only feeds the host (us), it also feeds the microbiome, improves our immune function, the production of essential vitamins and hormones; and, how these beneficial bacteria improve our overall health.

Dr. Kevin Hall spoke about The Calculus of Calories and discussed how maintaining a healthy weight is not just about calories; it has even more to do with the composition of the food eaten and how this affects our metabolism. He explained how changing the composition of the diet affects calorie burning and fat storage. He discussed how a decrease in the intake of simple carbohydrates and increasing the consumption of healthy fats positively affects the insulin level, calorie burning and fat metabolism.

Dr. Xiao Ou Shu, of Vanderbilt University, reviewed the clinical research on soy products and breast cancer. She explained how the type of estrogen in soy products actually appears to be protective against breast cancer and sited several studies done in Japan and in the U.S. This is a significant topic since so many women have decreased their consumption of meat by eating more soy-based protein and want to know that this is a healthier option. According to Dr. Xiao, the research does support this.

Caroline Trapp's lecture focused on de-prescribing insulin. She advocates decreasing, reducing or not prescribing insulin in the first place. She reported on many patients who had high blood sugar levels and how a lifestyle approach with healthy nutrition and exercise enabled some individuals to avoid starting insulin, while others were able to lower their levels or even discontinue insulin. I have reported the same results from many of my patients who followed the recommendations for a plant-based nutrition program combined with exercise and weight reduction. She discussed one patient who lost almost 300 pounds with this approach and then actually introduced him to the 700 attendees as he was sitting in the audience! He stood up and got a standing ovation — that was the most emotional part of the conference.

Next, Jim Stevenson from the University of Southampton discussed the attention deficit hyperactivity disorder (ADHD). This appears to be related to not only nutrition but also to genetic differences, alcohol and tobacco use by the mother before the child is born, low birth weight and high lead exposure. He talked about nutrition of the mother prenatally as well as nutrition of the child. Exposure of the child to foods with pesticides, food colorings and other additives appeared to be related to the incidence of ADHD. In

Europe, there is a warning label on foods with artificial colors and several candy manufacturers have voluntarily removed them from their products. Although the research is not as clear, many parents believe their child's behavior is related to eating foods with sugar and when they eliminate sugar from the child's diet, their ADHD symptoms decline. One nutritional treatment thought to be helpful is fish oil. Since we know that free fatty acids in fish oil are good for the brain, the addition of fish/fish oil to the diet sounds useful for many reasons.

Jae Hee Kang, from Brigham and Women's Hospital, noted that by 2050 the incidence of Alzheimer's Dementia (AD) will double with an estimated cost of $1 trillion! From 2000 until 2013 the incidence of deaths related to AD increased 70%. We know that the risk increases with age; however, it also increases with excess alcohol use, lower educational level and by any other mechanism which interferes with blood flow to the brain. It is believed that antioxidants in fruits and vegetables decrease the risk for AD.

Dr. Neal Barnard, the President of Physicians Committee for Responsible Medicine (PCRM), ended the conference with an intriguing presentation on cheese addiction and the health implications of eating too much cheese. This was a fascinating presentation since he presented the science behind food addiction and the clinical implications of eating a food product that is 70% fat. This is also a food loaded with salt, calories and no fiber. In 1909, the average American ate 3.8 lbs. of cheese annually; in 2013 that number was up to 33 lbs. With that increase we have also seen an increase in the rate of obesity, heart disease, diabetes and many other chronic illnesses which have been described by many as Western diseases. Dr. Barnard also discussed the relationship of a high-fat diet and hormonal problems, prostate cancer and osteoporosis.

At the end of his lecture, and most of the other presentations, the speakers brightened up the day by reporting the clinical, scientific evidence-based solution to most of the health problems facing Americans today – food! Yes, food is the cause of most health problems in America and healthy nutrition is the cure! For two days and 16 hours of lectures those of us sitting in the audience heard repeatedly that healthy eating lowers the risk of chronic disease and cancer, improves the quality of lives and even extends lifespan — what an easy way to live better!

- Dr. Sal

5-2-1-0+9 is a Healthy Equation!

5-2-1-0+9 is a healthy equation! My daughter has heard me mention this equation many times and she now understands its significance in her life — she even explains it to others! In our home we talk a lot about things that keep a person healthy and things we do that can make us sick. We remind each other how important our health is and what can happen if our health fails. We do our best to stick to the numbers.

This equation is used as a reminder to focus on five behaviors which, if done consistently, result in above average health. Starting with 5, this number reminds us to eat at least 5 servings of vegetables and fruits daily. Notice the order of the wording: vegetables and fruits, not fruits and vegetables, which is the way most people recite this phrase. I specifically focus on the order because healthy nutrition is attained when eating more vegetables than fruits. The problem with eating too many fruits is sugar. The epidemic of diabetes, pre-diabetes and obesity in the world today is the direct result of sugar overload. In addition to these illnesses, sugar in excess also increases the risk for cardiovascular disease and Alzheimer's dementia which is now called Type 3 diabetes because of the way the excess sugar affects the brain. When you eat more vegetables than fruits, especially organic, you get more vitamins, minerals, antioxidants and fiber. All of these nutrients are what keep the body fueled and ready to go! Vegetables are low in calories, low in fat and high in nutrition. They are also very filling. When you eat lots of bulky food, the stomach gets filled and sends messages to the brain saying, "I'm full – don't eat anymore!" This is a great way to maintain a healthy body weight. It is important to eat at least 5 servings of vegetables a day and 1-2 fruits to add more fiber that is beneficial for the function of the gastrointestinal tract. Without enough fiber, a person is at risk for chronic constipation and, over a long period of time, this increases a person's risk for many different bowel illnesses.

The number 2 refers to no more than two hours of screen time per day. This is time spent in front of the computer, tablet, TV and phone. If you count the number of minutes in a day (1440) and realize that 7-8 hours are spent sleeping, 5-6 hours are spent in school and then 2 hours sitting in front of a screen playing games, the child spends most of their day sedentary. This is not healthy. It is no wonder we have an epidemic of childhood obesity in this country. As parents, we must encourage our children to go out and play and we must go out with them! This is good for our health while bonding with our children. The author, John Maxwell, writes: "if you want to know what's important to a person, look to see how he spends his time and money." When we spend time with our children, we are telling them they are important to us. Get off the couch, go outside, run around with your children and have fun!

The next number is 1 and relates to exercise. We must encourage our children to get one hour of physical activity daily. There is no better way to keep the heart and vascular system healthy. Research teaches us that cardiovascular disease starts very early in life. Autopsies from many of the men and women who died in previous wars revealed early arteriosclerosis (hardening of the arteries) in 18- and 20-year-old adults. Research also shows us that exercise is a preventive measure that wards off vascular disease. Again, one hour of physical activity daily for children and adults!

The number 0 refers to zero sugary drinks. Yes, zero! In order to define a sugary drink, you must read the label because it is not only soda that is a sugary drink. A typical 8 oz. glass of cow's milk contains 16 grams of sugar – that is 4 teaspoons! The general recommendation is to get no more than 9 teaspoons of sugar per day from everything you eat and drink. If you then have a glass of sweet tea or an energy drink later in the day, you are over the limit. Do not think diet sodas are any healthier because the no-calorie sweetener, Aspartame, in diet drinks and foods is digested into formaldehyde (embalming fluid!).

When you look at the weight of the U.S. population since diet sodas were introduced, the average weight has actually increased, and the health of the population overall has declined significantly. So...no sugary drinks allowed! If your children like milk, give them unsweetened almond, soy or rice milk. They can get these healthier alternatives in school simply by asking for them.

The number 9 is added to remind us that children need 9 hours of sleep nightly. Just as we set an alarm clock to get up in the morning, we should have a defined time to get the children to bed ensuring they get enough quality sleep. None of us can be fully healthy without enough sleep, especially growing children. Help your children wind down at the end of the day by turning the lights lower, getting the house cool and quiet and having them do relaxing activities. A dark room is necessary for the brain to make growth hormone, essential for normal growth and development.

The equation **5-2-1-0+9** sets up a great foundation of healthy living for our children and the entire family. We can use this equation for adults with some modification. For many adults, computers are a large part of their work day. The number 2 is used as a reminder for adults to limit the non-work screen time to no more than two hours per day. Otherwise, we can use the same equation for adults. I encourage parents to go online and print out the **5-2-1-0+9** flyer and hang it on your refrigerator as a daily reminder to the family. Next, talk about the importance of all these elements when sitting at the dinner table for a healthy meal. Having the entire family engaged is a great way to keep everyone healthy!

- Dr. Sal

Vo2 as a Risk Factor for Cardiovascular Disease

The most common cause of death and disability in the U.S. and most developed countries is cardiovascular disease (CVD). This includes heart attacks, congestive heart failure, high blood pressure, high cholesterol, strokes and possibly even dementia. Risk factors for CVD include smoking, male gender, a family history of premature CVD, sedentary lifestyle, high-blood pressure, high cholesterol and certainly unhealthy eating. When looking at the risk related to a sedentary lifestyle, we find this correlates directly with what is defined as low-aerobic capacity. Exercise tolerance can be measured by a number known as Vo2, the ability of the body to use oxygen. When exercising, the muscles function well only as long as oxygen and other nutrients are available. When the level of exercise exceeds the body's ability to deliver the necessary oxygen and nutrients, the muscles begin to fatigue and cramp. This is the point where the individual should stop the exercise.

In an article in the *European Journal of Preventive Cardiology*, researchers looked at various risk factors for CVD including smoking, high blood pressure, high cholesterol and Vo2 (aerobic capacity). They had a representative sample of men born in 1913 and followed them from 50-99 years of age. At age 54, 792 men performed an ergometer exercise test; 656 were able to complete the test to a maximum level. These individuals were then followed for another 45 years. The results showed that Vo2 was a significant predictor of mortality, independent of other risk factors such a smoking, high blood pressure and high cholesterol. From this study it was felt that adding information from the exercise test improved risk prediction; that is, the ability to identify those who will suffer a heart attack, a stroke or early

180

death because of CVD. A previous study followed people for 10-15 years and another for 26 years. The current study followed these individuals for 45 years! If the readers want to delve into it in more detail, it is *The Study of Men Born in 1913*.

Exercise-stress testing provides information more than just the Vo2 number. It allows the physician to measure the maximum workload of the heart, the ability of the heart to recover after maximum exercise and the response of the blood pressure to exercise. In addition, the physician is able to look at the heart rate and blood pressure at four minutes after exercise. This is when the heart rate and blood pressure should be back to normal for the individual. When it takes the heart a longer time to recover, the physician knows that this person's heart is more at risk for cardiovascular complications.

The study also reported hazard regression rates, the statistical numbers that relate a measurement to the rate of a negative health consequence. The data for hazard rates shows that for every increase in Vo2 (aerobic capacity) the death rate from all causes decreases. Conversely, death rates rose with increases in body weight, blood pressure, cholesterol and smoking. This study was summarized as follows: during 45 years of follow up, low aerobic capacity (Vo2) was associated with higher all-cause mortality in middle-aged men, independent of traditional cardiovascular risk factors. The last part of this sentence is important. The most common risk factors used to help identify people at risk for CVD include those mentioned above (high blood pressure, cholesterol, body weight and smoking). Exercise tolerance is not generally part of the risk factors; this study indicates it should be as it adds significant information to the person's risk profile.

When the physician itemizes a person's risk factors for CVD, they help the person understand what might happen in the next five to ten years in relation to cardiovascular health. The Framingham Risk Score uses information such as blood pressure, cholesterol, smoking history and other details to calculate a ten-year risk of a heart attack.

By adding a Vo2 measurement to these traditional risk factors, the physician is able to give the person more information about their risk.

This study shows that as the Vo2 improves, the risk for heart attacks and strokes decreases. The American Heart Association recommends at least 30 minutes of moderately intense exercise most days of the week. Exercise is part of the foundation for healthy living and fitful aging. At the Healthy Life Centers, the exercise specialists perform aerobic capacity (Vo2) tests. I often add this to the tests for my patients since it gives me and the patient more information about their overall health. We can then develop an action plan to reduce risk factors and improve overall health. The goal is to enable the individual to live a healthier, longer life.

In summary, exercise is a significant part of the foundation for healthy living. Before starting a formal exercise program, I recommend checking with your physician or health care provider. Schedule an exercise test that will indicate if your heart is ready for exercise. It will also give you the Vo2 number described above. This number may be used as the baseline. After exercising for a time period, repeat the test to see how you have improved. Compare that number to someone your age or younger using these numbers to tweak your exercise routine. Exercise and healthy nutrition are the keys to staying young and enjoying a fit-full life!

- Dr. Sal

Medical Students are Champions for Lifestyle Medicine

S tudents at the Heritage College of Osteopathic Medicine in Ohio are champions for Lifestyle Medicine! Recently I had the honor of speaking there about the Food is Medicine program we have been working on at Lee Health [in Fort Myers, FL] since 2010. My focus was on the science of nutrition supporting the use of food to help people prevent, treat and reverse chronic Illness.

Many medical students made me aware of the lifestyle medicine club they developed; and, how excited they were to hear about alternative ways to help patients. The students were primarily first and second year medical students and their enthusiasm was infectious! The majority of the students appeared to be in good physical health, trim and fit. Many brought their lunch and I was pleased to see the salads, hummus and fruits.   I spoke with the student who started the lifestyle medicine club to discover she recently completed the Boston Marathon and runs 5k races in 19 minutes, an amazingly fast time. As such, I was tremendously pleased to know that these future physicians are personally and professionally engaged in wellness. Later I presented my *Food is Medicine* lecture to a group of physicians, dietitians, other health care professionals and community leaders. After eating a scrumptious plant-based meal, we discussed the need for changing the current health care system from the sick care system into a system which promotes health and wellness.

Personally, I am pleased to be part of a system of health care which has progressed over the past 100 years as evidenced by the advancement of surgical procedures, pharmaceuticals and medical treatments, which cure many sicknesses. Despite all this, the health of Americans has declined dramatically in recent years. Approximately

70% of the chronic illnesses people suffer from today are due to unhealthy lifestyle behaviors. Only a small percentage of the population get the necessary minutes of exercise daily, eat the recommended number of servings of vegetables and fruits and do not smoke. Many in the U.S. do not place health as their first priority. Only when health fails, or someone is diagnosed with cancer or a chronic illness, do they wake up to realize that good health should not be taken for granted.

This is the best time for students to be involved in health care. There is a movement across the country transitioning our sick care system into a health care system, helping people become and stay healthy.

The goal is to help people avoid disease and disability — this is where lifestyle medicine shines! The evolution of lifestyle medicine has come about because the current system of health care is not sustainable. Most of our population is unhealthy. In America we spend more per capita on health care than any other country in the world yet we are far down the list of the healthiest countries. Our standard of living leads us to spend the last years of our lives in sickness, not wellness. This is in contrast to people who live in Blue Zones®, the places in the world where folks live beyond 100 years of age. The lifestyle behaviors of these folks have been extensively researched; from this study we know these people eat natural foods, stay active daily and have good social support. They have a purpose in life and contribute to family and community, despite their advanced age. These people grow old with vitality and die of old age, not because they develop chronic disease or cancer as many do in the U.S.

Lifestyle is the key to longevity. It's the reason many people get sick and the reason many people remain healthy. We must decide the type of lifestyle we will live. The science of lifestyle medicine supports the following as the foundation for healthy living: eating non-processed and natural foods, being active, getting the required number of minutes of formal exercise including weight lifting, minimizing stress and getting seven to eight hours of quality sleep nightly, and having a purpose in life. When life has meaning and we focus on being healthy, we make the world a better place — everyone benefits!

- Dr. Sal

Corporate Cuisine

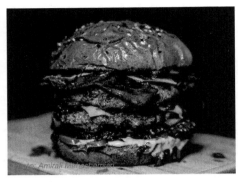

A while ago I wrote about the U.S. government banning imports and exports of ivory from African elephants in an effort to protect this endangered animal. My question is … why is our government not protecting the health of what could be considered another endangered species — our children?

For the past six years, I have been researching the link between food, health and disease, looking at the food served in our elementary and high schools; and, wondering why we continue to feed our children disease-promoting foods. Further research into this topic reveals massive financial subsidies by the government for foods such as pepperoni pizza, chicken nuggets, hot dogs and cow's milk. In addition to the subsidies, food and beverage companies spent $149 million marketing such foods in elementary and high schools! All these efforts have led to a massive increase in rates of obesity and diabetes, facts many continue to ignore. Since 1980 the number of obese children has doubled, while the number of obese adolescents has increased four times! We have created massive health problems in this country as a result of corporate greed. The resulting sobering statistic is that the next generation is thought by many to have a shorter life expectancy than the previous. Certainly, this generation will be sicker, have a lower quality of life; and, spend more money on health care.

The substandard meals in our schools are, in large part, due to excessive lobbying in order to influence governmental policies overseeing the school lunch program. A recent article written about

186

milk money stated that food service in the U.S. is a complex series of government and corporate partnerships which support Big Ag or agribusiness. The relationship between these companies and the USDA focuses efforts more on corporate profits rather than the health of the children they are supposed to protect and serve. While many schools have such limited financial support, they request school supplies from the teachers and parents of the students. These companies are spending millions to advertise and promote the consumption of unhealthy food.

The original school lunch program was started around the time of the Great Depression when poor children were becoming malnourished. In 1945, President Truman signed the National School Lunch Act, giving rise to formation of the National School Lunch Program. Over the subsequent years, budget cuts forced the outsourcing of meals that were previously hand made in the schools. These budget cuts resulted in a significant decline in the quality of the food, making it apparent that the health of the students eating the food was not the main concern. Today, many school meals are supplied by major corporations such as Chick-fil-A, Domino's, Subway, Tyson foods, Pizza Hut and McDonald's. Currently, 31 million students receive free lunch in more than 100,000 schools across the nation.

When it comes to the control these companies have over the school lunch program, look no further than the dairy industry. Despite the fact that many children are either lactose intolerant or allergic to cow's milk, access to dairy-free milk had been denied due to the marketing efforts of a division of the USDA known as DMI (Dairy Management, Inc.). The focus of this department is to increase the amount of dairy consumed. Marketing campaigns such as *Got Milk?* and *Beef: It's What's for Dinner* provide $557 million to promote meat, egg and dairy sales in comparison to $51 million to promote the consumption of vegetables and fruits.

Even pressure from the former First Lady Michelle Obama did not make a significant impact. She started an initiative called the

Healthy, Hunger-Free Kids Act to raise the nutritional profile of school lunches. When there was disagreement regarding two tablespoons of tomato paste on pizza counting as a serving of vegetable, more than a dozen food companies attempted to protect the profits of the $450 million made for supplying pizzas to schools. They created the Coalition for Sustainable School Meals to fight the changes attempted by Mrs. Obama and unfortunately, they won. Lobbyists (both Republicans and Democrats) including a senator from the state which was home to one of the largest suppliers of pizza to schools worked to defeat this initiative. Big money won the fight at the expense of the health of our children!

Currently, most school meals exceed the recommended limits for fat, salt and sugar; and, if students are not learning about healthy nutrition in school and not getting this most important education at home — how do we break the cycle? In New York, the Coalition for Healthy School Food created the *Cool School Food Program* to deal with this. They tested pilot programs using plant-based, whole food recipes in school cafeterias. The goal is to change the thinking of students, parents, school administrators; and, local/national governments to change the culture surrounding the school lunch programs. Only by relentless commitment will we transform the health of our children by improving the nutrition served in our school systems. We can no longer be ignorant to the blatant disregard agribusiness has for the health of our children and the nation. It is time to stop accepting these abuses and insist on healthy food for our children and ourselves. As a nation, we must make health the number one priority!

- Dr. Sal

How Is Your Energy Level?

When you get up in the morning, how is your energy level? Is it good enough so that you are able to get out of bed relatively quickly, ready to start the day, or do you drag yourself out of bed looking immediately for that first cup of coffee?

Energy production is one of the body's most important biologic functions. In relation to how energy is produced, it is one of the most misunderstood. This is evident when reading the content of so-called energy drinks that are essentially loaded with caffeine and sugar. It is important to understand how energy is produced and how to make more of it.

In every cell of the body there are energy producing units called mitochondria. These are the specialized portions of the cells which make ATP, the chemical equivalent of what we know to be energy. When a certain amount of glucose and fatty acids enter the mitochondria, they are used to make ATP; this is what drives all chemical reactions in the body. Without ATP, the trillions of cells in the body are not able to carry out their normal functions.

There is a misconception on how we can make more energy; this usually involves more caffeine, sugar and stimulants — none of which actually work in the long run. Certainly, in the short time period after having an energy drink, the body feels more energetic because of the effects caffeine, sugar and other stimulants have on the heart. They speed up the heart and increases blood pressure. The added sugar increases insulin which drives more glucose into the cells. For a short time, the person feels more energetic, yet in a few hours, they start to crash. When the effects of the caffeine and sugar wear off, the sugar level plummets, the person feels tired again, might

189

actually feel jittery and start thinking about the need for another energy drink.

Instead of reaching for the typical energy drinks, a person wanting more energy should eat and drink nutritious foods that are easy to digest and help to produce the ATP necessary. The definition of nutritious should be foods and drinks that are natural, non-toxic, with the proper balance of healthy protein, fats and carbohydrates. In today's world of diets which are supposed to make people into athletes and super-models, many people avoid major food groups and carbohydrates. Others stay on super low-fat diets and eat so much protein that their kidneys are compromised.

The three major food categories necessary for good health are fats, proteins and carbohydrates. All are needed for the body to carry out its normal, physiologic functions. Limiting fats too much interferes with normal brain function, decreases the production of vital hormones, and, makes cell membranes less healthy. Limiting healthy carbohydrates makes it harder for the cells to make ATP, for the reasons detailed above. Eating too much protein damages the kidneys over time and is unnecessary. For the average person, the need for protein is about 60-70 grams per day. One cup of lentils provides 18 grams — it does not require a lot of food to supply the daily requirement of protein.

Avocados, walnuts, flax seed and salmon are examples of healthy fats. Fruits provide good carbohydrates and fiber necessary to keep the GI tract healthy. If a person wants to juice their fruits, it is more beneficial to do this in a blender as it retains all the fiber. Using a juicer removes fiber and produces a glass of pure sugar which overwhelms the body's ability to handle glucose. Whatever sugar (glucose) in the bloodstream is not used for energy is converted into fat and becomes stored in the liver, around the heart, under the skin of the abdomen, buttocks and hips.

Protein is the other issue. Protein intake is necessary on a daily basis since our body does not store protein as it does fats and carbohydrates, therefore, a daily supply is necessary but must be provided in a level that is healthy, not harmful. Protein sources include all animal meats, dairy, soy products, beans, nuts and vegetables. Not all proteins are alike, because of the contaminants in many sources of protein. Unfortunately, the meats available today are not the same quality as the meats our grandparents ate. Animals then were raised on farms, eating grass and enjoying a relatively stress-free life in the sunshine. Today, animals are raised in confined, animal-feeding operations (CAFO). Thousands are raised in such close quarters they do not have enough room to move, do not see sunlight, are majorly stressed and for most of their lives stand in their own feces. For more on this topic read, *The Meaty Truth*, an eye-opening book detailing the realities of how many of the foods Americans consume may cause the majority of chronic illnesses and cancers. Calorie for calorie, vegetables are a healthier source of protein and when buying organic and non-GMO, contaminants that destroy health are avoided.

Vitamins and minerals round out the discussion on healthy eating and energy production. The macro molecules (proteins, fats and carbohydrates) are the components needed for cells to perform their vital functions. Cells cannot do this without vitamins and minerals which are needed to perform all the thousands of required chemical reactions.

In addition to the nutrients needed to produce ATP/energy, the body needs seven to eight hours of quality sleep, as well as stress management. When a person is chronically stressed, they have an elevated level of cortisol. This is the stress hormone which interferes with many vital functions and in time lessens the quality and length of one's life.

In summary, if you want to be full of energy, supply the body with nutritious food and drink, get enough sleep nightly, take vitamins/ supplements when needed and manage stress. If possible, take a 10-

minute afternoon power nap and have a vegetable smoothie, both will do the body more good than any energy drink on the market!

- Dr. Sal

The Choices We Make

Because I love to read, over the years I have probably read thousands of books, many more articles and research papers. Since I am in the medical field, most of my reading has been health related, although, I have read almost every business book written by John Maxwell. A recent article that I found intriguing is, *Analysis & Valuation of Health & Climate Change Co-benefits of Dietary Change*. The article focuses on the duel health and environmental benefits of reducing the amount of animal foods in our diet. The purpose of this research was to quantify the link between health and environmental consequences of dietary change. This article was fascinating to me especially after recently reading, *The Meaty Truth*, by Shushana Castle. This book is filled with much data regarding the health, economic and planetary consequences of agribusiness. The article focuses on the beneficial consequences of a change in our dietary consumption. If we love ourselves, our children, the community and planet we live on, this article and book contain facts we cannot ignore. I encourage everyone to read both.

Because writing, talking and discussing food is extremely emotional, know I am only the messenger. Everyone should know the facts and health implications regarding the food they eat, realizing that many of the facts about agribusiness are not known to the general public. Much information is purposely withheld from public consumption since knowing and understanding the raw details of food processing would disgust most people and would make many look for healthier sources of food. In my years of practicing medicine, I have seen many people suffer and die from food related illnesses — this situation is only getting worse. Over 30% of the population is now

193

obese and over 60% overweight. We have an epidemic of diabetes in adults and now diagnose adult-onset diabetes in adolescents! The rates of heart disease and strokes are staggering, while Alzheimer's dementia is destroying the lives of many individuals and families. Although President Nixon declared a war on cancer in the 1980s, we are losing the war. The sad truth is that the majority of chronic illnesses and common cancers are due to the foods we eat and, the lifestyles we live. Even sadder is the fact that most of these health problems are avoidable. We have the power to change ourselves, our community and our planet. This is what the above mentioned article and book detail so eloquently.

The article details how small changes in the consumption of animal products (meat and dairy) could have tremendous benefits in global health, by reducing emissions of carbon dioxide which produces global warming and create widespread positive changes for the planet. The authors calculate the number of avoided deaths and the number of years of life saved. Shushana Castle's book details how changes in what we eat would affect the billions of animals slaughtered annually, decrease the need to get rid of millions of pounds of manure that pollutes our planet, decrease the risk of antibiotic resistance, stop the massive deforestation, significantly decrease health care costs and improve the lives of millions!

The current generation of adults is tremendously unhealthy yet even more important is the fact that we are growing the next generation to be even less healthy and with a shorter lifespan! We are teaching our children by our actions and inactions that eating unhealthy food is acceptable. We are not teaching them to live healthy lives and mature into healthy, productive adults. We are giving them the message that it is acceptable to abuse animals, neglect our environment and destroy the planet. We must focus on what life will be like with many unforeseen health problems — a world that has been decimated.

Because the health status of our population and the health problems we deal with are getting worse, I believe it is necessary to be blunt. We need to be aware of our food sources before getting to our dinner table. It is time to make significant changes in the way we eat, exercise and live. There is no time to waste!

Healthy Lee of Lee County in Fort Myers, Florida is a community-wide initiative designed to improve the health of the population in Lee County, Florida. The goal is to improve access to parks and places to exercise, making healthy food available and affordable, educating school children in all aspects of healthy living and changing policies to improve the health of everyone. I encourage the reader to get involved and become part of the solution. The choices made today will significantly affect our lives and the lives of our children for years to come. Thanks to all the devoted people who work diligently every day to make this a reality.

- Dr. Sal

Adherence to Lifestyle Guidelines Decreases Risk of Cancer

A recent study published in the *British Journal of Nutrition* analyzed how lifestyle behaviors affected the risk of cancer in healthy, premenopausal women. For cancer prevention, the World Cancer Research Fund (WCRF) and the American Institute for Cancer Research (AICR) recommend eight lifestyle behaviors shown to lower the risk of cancer: no smoking, maintaining a lean body mass (measured as BMI/body mass index), minimizing the consumption of calorie-rich foods such as sodas, red and processed meats, limiting alcohol, participating in regular physical activity and consuming a plant-based diet.

The researchers evaluated the adherence to these recommendations and compared these rates to three biomarkers of oxidation and inflammation: the levels of Vitamin E, F2 isoprostane, and C-reactive protein (CRP). Oxidation is a chemical process that occurs in cells, described as rusting of the cells from within. When specific toxins/toxic situations affect the cells of the body, the cells become injured and start to oxidize. As a result, the cells are unable to function normally; and, depending on the organ this occurs in, certain diseases/cancers may develop. When this appears in the arteries of the body, the individual develops arteriosclerosis or hardening of the arteries. This leads to high blood pressure, blockage of the normal blood flow, increases the risk for strokes, heart attacks and heart failure. When the body experiences high levels of oxidation, it produces more vitamin E (an antioxidant) to combat this condition. The C-reactive protein test is a measure of inflammation in the body and the F2-isoprostane test is another measure of oxidation. These tests give the researcher information about the person's internal

196

response to external factors such as smoking, lack of exercise and a high fat diet.

Smoking has direct effects on blood vessels and causes endothelial dysfunction. The hundreds of toxic chemicals in cigarette smoke directly damage the lining cells of the arteries and may cause the person many different cardiovascular problems as well as many cancers. The World Health Organization (WHO) developed a position statement which clearly warned the general public about the significant dangers of red and processed meats (bacon, sausage, lunch meats) and specifically warned of the increased risk of cancer, especially colon cancer. High calorie foods contribute to weight gain, obesity, diabetes and other illnesses. Soda and other sweet drinks increase the risk for diabetes, obesity, metabolic syndrome, cardiovascular disease, Alzheimer's dementia and more. In addition to what the cancer organizations recommend against, they also advise exercising, maintaining a normal body weight and eating more plant-based foods.

When the researchers studied individuals with high adherence rates to these recommendations, they found those who followed most of the recommendations had the lowest rates of the three biomarkers (CRP, Vitamin E and F2-isoprostane) — meaning they had the lowest levels of oxidation and inflammation. Overall, they were healthier and had a lower risk for future cancer. The exact title of the article I am referring to is, *Adherence to Cancer Prevention Recommendations and Antioxidant and Inflammatory Status in Premenopausal Women*.

These are recommendations I make to all my patients, family and friends. Often these recommendations are met with resistance and comments about being too radical. My response...having a stroke, heart bypass surgery or chemotherapy for cancer is radical! When an individual follows most of the recommendations listed as guidelines by these cancer societies, they become healthier, enjoy life and live longer. When the same individual does not follow these guidelines,

197

they are less healthy, have an increased risk, may suffer from chronic disease or cancer, live a poorer quality and a shorter life.

Most of what happens regarding our health as we age is a matter of choice…adhere to recommendations that will afford better health or ignore the guidelines and travel down the road that many in America travel – the road to sickness, disability, disease and early death. The American way of life is unhealthy. We spend more money on health care than any other country in the world; yet we have some of the worst health problems. In 2019, the U.S. was #35 on the list, meaning that 35 other countries were healthier than us despite the fact that we spend more money on health care than any other country in the world! Those are sobering statistics.

We must do something about this…follow the guidelines, live better and longer. Guard your health like it is your most prized possession, because it is!

- Dr. Sal

Do Not Hold Back!

A visit with your physician should be a comfortable experience. At times there are issues a person wants to talk about yet the topic is embarrassing and the conversation never begins. When this happens, everyone loses. As the title of this article states, don't hold back! The reason for visiting with your physician/health care provider is to tell them what is going on, how you are feeling and describe symptoms that will lead them to a diagnosis. No symptom or complaint is too trivial to discuss.

Something might sound trivial to the layperson yet to the physician's ear it may help identify a significant problem. A person might complain of heartburn and when questioned further, this symptom may actually be angina – chest pain related to poor circulation in the arteries of the heart. If the physician asks, when does this heartburn occur and the patient's response is when I exercise, immediately the physician knows this is more likely heart related and not a GI problem. I recommend my patients keep a list of health concerns occurring between visits and bring the list to the next visit. Also, I ask them to write down questions and concerns to address. If time does not allow us to get through the entire list, we reschedule another visit to finish. Lastly, patients are encouraged to email me with non-urgent questions. In my office we use an electronic system called EPIC MY Chart that allows for additional communication and even allows a patient to access parts of their medical record. The goal is for the patient to become and stay well; these additional methods of communication help achieve this.

Complaints or symptoms that initially appear too embarrassing to bring up, are not! One common complaint is constipation. This is a significant health issue since chronic constipation interferes at times with activities in daily living, however, it may increase the risk for life-threatening illnesses such as colitis or even colon cancer. There are many reasons for chronic constipation including not drinking enough water, eating enough fiber or getting enough exercise. The standard American diet lends itself to more problems with bowel movements. When toxins persist in the colon, and there are dozens of toxins found in the standard American foods, this increases the risk and incidence of inflammation within the GI tract, increasing the occurrence of long term various GI problems as mentioned above. Chronic constipation also negatively affects the microbiome, the environment within the GI tract and colon where bacteria reside. Chronic constipation can alter the beneficial bacteria in the colon and allow the growth of harmful bacteria. If this happens, a person may develop alternating constipation and diarrhea. This may also affect the natural production of vitamins, the absorption of nutrients and the ability to maintain a normal body weight.

Another complaint often thought too embarrassing to mention is erectile dysfunction (ED). This is a common male health problem. Decreased libido also affects many females and should be discussed. There are many reasons for ED as well as deceased libido. Some are physical, some chemical, others hormonally related and can even occur as a result of psychological problems, stress or induced by a prescription medication. Cardiovascular disease (CVD) is the number one cause of illness and early death in the United States. Often, ED is the first sign of CVD – the "canary in the coal mine" as the saying goes. After the individual opens the discussion, the cause must be determined. The physician will look for signs of poor circulation, test for diabetes, review the person's medications and ask questions about smoking, alcohol or other lifestyle behaviors which might help identify the reason for the ED or decreased libido. The health care provider will also help the patient understand there are many things that can be done to improve these complaints. Psychological support is very important when dealing with such sensitive issues.

Thinning hair is often another concern that is not initially discussed, even though the individual is bothered by this. Again, nothing is too embarrassing to discuss with your physician or health care provider. That is what they are there for – to help with any concerns, health issues and questions. A person might think they have one problem, yet find when they describe their symptoms to their physician, a completely different diagnosis is made. Depression is a good example. I have seen many people complaining of chronic fatigue or persistent aches and pains. They believe they have fibromyalgia or chronic fatigue syndrome, anemia or thyroid problems. In reality, they are depressed. There are times a person knows they are depressed and hesitates to bring it up, believing there is a stigma attached to this diagnosis. As the conversation opens up, I assure my patients there is nothing to be embarrassed about if they are depressed, anxious or stressed. The workup might reveal a chemical or hormonal imbalance, a post-traumatic stress disorder, associated with chronic sleep deprivation or be the side effect of a prescription medication being used for another health problem. Talking through these issues, allows the physician to establish a list of possible health problems before arriving at a specific diagnosis.

No problem is too small to discuss with your health care provider; bringing up all symptoms or concerns usually results in better short and long-term health. When health is the number one priority, all other goals are achievable.

- Dr. Sal

201

Adding Complementary to Traditional Medicine

Is there anything that can be added to traditional medical care to improve health and wellness? Do we as health care providers know enough about complementary and alternative medicine that would add benefits to traditional medical care? In training or our practice, have we learned enough about the impact of food, exercise and lifestyle on the risk and incidence of disease and how healthy nutrition impacts both? Are health care providers clear on the definition of healthy nutrition?

In the last 50 years we have seen tremendous advances in pharmaceuticals, surgical procedures and other aspects of medical care while the health of the population declines as more people suffer from chronic illness, cancer and other debilitating diseases. Much of the decline in health comes as a result of unhealthy processed food, agribusiness, a tremendous reliance on prescription medications and an extremely sedentary population. The majority of people in the U.S. do not eat the recommended number of vegetables and fruits daily and they do not get the recommended number of minutes of exercise daily. Many people still smoke cigarettes despite the warnings. More now are switching to e-cigarettes assuming this is a healthier alternative (NOT!). Many do not see their physician for regular check-ups and when they do, the results of their blood pressure, cholesterol and other markers of health, are not in the goal range. Overall, lifestyles in the U.S. have declined rapidly over the last 50 years, not only contributing to but actually causing, many of the health problems people suffer from daily.

There is hope and there are solutions! We must make adjustments in how we live and think about medical care. When I do public presentations, I ask the audience, "When you have high blood pressure and go to the doctor, what happens?" The answer usually is, "A prescription is written." Usually the same goes for high cholesterol and many other medical problems. This statement is intended in no way to demean traditional medical care. I still write many prescriptions and have practiced traditional medical care for over 20 years. This statement is made to emphasize the point that we should first consider the cause of the problem and then decide if the individual is able to make any lifestyle changes to correct it. If we look at the cause for high blood pressure and high cholesterol, we often find the individual is living a lifestyle that at least significantly contributes to the problem. If we are able to eliminate the cause, which may be a high-salt diet, lots of fatty foods or lack of exercise, we might alleviate the problem and avoid medication. In my clinical practice, I have found this approach works in many cases by not exposing the individual to the possible side effects of medications. I usually ask my patients, "Do you want to commit yourself to a lifetime of medication, as well as the expense, when the problem can be solved with a change in lifestyle?" In most cases, people like this approach and find that it does work.

Certainly, if this approach does not bring about the needed change in blood pressure or cholesterol, we have the benefit of medication and other therapies that traditional health care offers.

This approach should not be termed "alternative," but instead should be called "complementary" since that is what it is: all the non-traditional methods of treating and reversing disease complementing what can be done on the traditional side of medical care. These are the lifestyle approaches to health and well-being. We must be further educated in these complementary approaches to disease. It is important to understand and use the power of lifestyle medicine which in many cases works as well — or even better than prescriptions, procedures and surgeries!

As health care providers, we need to help our patients develop a healthy lifestyle action plan then help them monitor the effectiveness of lifestyle approaches adding these to the methods in our traditional doctor bags.

- Dr. Sal

What Is Health?

When asked the question: what is health, often the answer is, "the absence of disease." Is health really just the absence of disease or is it more than that? Many people do believe health is the absence of disease as there are many Americans who, by various criteria, are unhealthy; while those who currently do not have a disease, believe they are healthy.

If we look at the life of an average person in the U.S., we see that as a result of the standard American lifestyle, signs of poor health start to develop early, sometimes as early as five or six years of age. Certainly, one of the most obvious signs of poor health is weight. We now see many young children who are either overweight, even obese. As a result of the obesity epidemic, we are now diagnosing type-2 diabetes in children and adolescents. In the past, this was a disease of adults. Weight problems are often the starting point when a person becomes unhealthy.

Yet, there are many individuals who are overweight without diabetes, heart, or other diseases and believe they are healthy. For the folks in my practice, I look for other signs of health, known as risk factors.

Risk factors for poor health include the following: a sedentary life: not eating the recommended five to nine servings of vegetables and fruits daily (mostly vegetables); smoking cigarettes; not getting seven to eight hours of quality sleep nightly; having a lot of unmanageable stress; not having good social/spiritual support; having high blood pressure, cholesterol or glucose in the blood; and many others. There are functional risk factors such as shortness of breath with minimal exertion and exercise intolerance. I am always concerned when a 50-year old tells me they are unable to climb a few flights of stairs or walk briskly without becoming short of breath. When a person describes a lifestyle that is functionally limited, I am concerned this person is not presently healthy and, they will become unhealthier in time.

In defining health, we should be looking at function and how well a person is aging as they advance in years. Being healthy is more about maintaining function, vitality, energy and a youthful spirit as the years increase. Let's compare a 75-year-old woman who is healthier than a 50-year-old man. The woman is independent, able to do most of the things she wants to physically, is mentally and cognitively well and looks forward to getting up each morning, to be a productive part of society. The 50-year-old man has a hard time running around with his children on the playground, flops on the couch after an eight-hour workday, has little desire to engage in social activities with family or friends and looks at each new day with a negative outlook.

Health is about mental and physical vitality. It is an energy that exudes from a person and is infectious to others. It is living life to the fullest and looking forward to each day with a sense of wanting to accomplish positive goals. It is being a productive part of family, work and community. It is being engaged and involved in life, doing things that make you happy and fulfilled.

The goal of the physician and other health care providers is to help people become and stay healthy. It is that simple. The hard part is doing it. This is where a team effort is required. The team includes each individual in combination with their physician/health care provider, the person's family and friends.

There is a saying, "you become who you associate with," and I believe this to be true. If you associate with people who enjoy being active and eating healthy food, have a positive outlook on life and are always willing to lend a hand to others then you will probably be more like them than someone with the opposite characteristics. As such, if you want to be healthy, make friends with healthy people. While this does not mean you should abandon all your unhealthy friends, if you want to attain a certain characteristic, you must know what it looks like. If you want to be healthy, see it in action!

In my practice I do many wellness exams. At the end of the visit I can tell them if they are healthy, have risk factors for disease, or have a diagnosis (a defined disease). The fewer the risk factors, the easier it is to tell a person they are healthy. When I hear a person describe their lifestyle of how active they are with enthusiasm and energy in their eyes and voice, I know this person is healthier than a person who portrays the opposite.

Once I understand the individual, I can work with them on a **Healthy Living Action Plan**. These daily priorities will continue to move the person toward better health. The foundation for the **Healthy Living Action Plan** is nutrition, physical activity, quality sleep, stress management, social and spiritual support, productivity and a sense of belonging. I also include giving back and paying it forward to remind others, as well as myself, there are always other individuals who have a tougher life than we do and we should help these folks when our paths cross.

An easy way to think about healthy eating is: *eat real food, not too much and mostly plants* (thanks to author, Michael Pollan, for this statement). With exercise, find every excuse to be active. Take the stairs instead of the elevator. Park far away from the store and walk. When golfing, forget the golf cart if you are allowed. With sleep, be sure to set an alarm clock to know when to go to bed ensuring at least seven hours of quality sleep nightly and — don't sweat the small stuff!

In summary, think of health certainly as the absence of disease but also as a state of functioning which allows you to do everything with abundant energy, vitality and a sense of purpose. Health is a journey rather than a place. We are all striving to get somewhere. With health, we are all striving to get to that place of goo, and even great, health.

- Dr. Sal

Doctor, How Do I Know If I Am Healthy?

Recently I received an e-mail from a gentleman who has been reading my articles asking, "What can a person in his 50s and 60s do to measure their vascular health when they appear healthy and have no indications of a health problem?" The reason he was asking this was because he believed he was in good health, eating an above-average diet, exercising and leading a stress-free life, only to find out that he had significant cardiac vascular disease (blockages in the arteries of the heart) requiring two stents. Interestingly, he had been monitoring his heart function while exercising using an app on his iPhone! His physician reviewed this information, sent him to a cardiologist who subsequently did a cardiac catheterization and found two areas of narrowing in the arteries of the heart. As a result of all this, the gentleman is now questioning how the situation developed when he had no previous indication (before the abnormalities showed up on his iPhone) of heart or vascular disease.

Since I began practicing internal medicine and now preventive health care, this story is not uncommon. Heart disease (vascular disease) is a slowly progressive process which occurs over years. It starts out as inflammation in the arteries, progresses to endothelial dysfunction. Plaque formation eventually disrupts the blood flow within the artery, causing heart muscle damage that can manifest as a heart attack, irregular heart rhythms or even heart failure. Inflammation occurs as a result of the American lifestyle: a high-fat diet, little exercise, lots of stress and poor sleep. This lifestyle causes inflammation in all the blood vessels from the brain to the feet and when inflammation continues, the process advances as described above. This process usually occurs slowly over years. As many

208

people age, they normally become less active and do not even notice any symptoms (such as poor exercise tolerance, shortness of breath or chest pain with exertion). They are not stressing the heart as they did when they were younger. Fortunately, this gentleman continued his exercise and noticed the problem on his iPhone which was monitoring his heart function.

The gentleman asked another good question, "How can you measure the health of your arteries at an early stage?" Many of the tests we use today identify late-stage vascular disease. A cardiac catheterization is an invasive test where a thin tube is passed into a large artery in the groin or in the arm and then passed into the main arteries of the heart. Images are then taken that show the main arteries to identify if there is any significant blockage. As described above, blockage seen via a catheterization is in the late stage of vascular disease. The question is: can we measure early disease, also known as endothelial dysfunction? Yes, there are blood tests which measure the inflammation in the arteries yet, they are relatively new tests. One is called CRP/C-reactive protein, a measure of inflammation. There are others such as MPO, Plac, oxidized LDL and F2-Isoprostane. None of these are routine tests and would be ordered if the physician suspects arterial inflammation. The diagnosis of arterial inflammation can be indirectly made when the physician sits with the patient and takes a history of how the individual lives. Their lifestyle will give the physician many clues this person probably has inflammation — it's all about lifestyle!

When a patient tells me, he has a good diet; I always ask specifically, "what do you eat for breakfast, lunch, dinner, snacks, etc.?" Also, "do you drink soda, sweet drinks and alcohol?" In addition, "how many minutes of exercise do you get daily and, in addition to aerobic (cardio) exercise, do you include any weight lifting?" I ask about sleep, stress and other life habits. All these questions provide information about whether the person has an inflammatory lifestyle.

In addition to taking a lifestyle history, the physician gets more information about the health of the vasculature from the physical examination, an EKG, blood pressure analysis and blood tests for cholesterol and blood sugar. When indicated, the individual might have an exercise stress test or possibly an echocardiogram, a two-dimensional picture of the heart measuring the heart pump function. Signs of poor health include hearing poor blood flow in the carotid arteries which supply the brain, listening with the stethoscope, hearing irregular heartbeats and diagnosing abnormalities on the EKG, stress test or ECHO.

When the physician gets an indication of inflammation, they will work with the patient to halt and hopefully reverse the progression. In general, this requires a significant change in lifestyle. A **healthy living action plan** needs to be developed. This starts with a nutrition plan to turn away from the standard American way of eating (the inflammatory diet). The individual is educated and, made to understand the importance of eating whole, unprocessed, nutritious foods. They learn about the importance of regular daily physical activity, stress management and quality sleep. They grow in their understanding that what you put in your body and what you do to your body results in either healthy aging … or disease, disability and decreased longevity.

The gentleman who wrote the e-mail wonders why there seems to be no early warning signs which identify disease. From the explanation above, you now know that is not true. There are many early warning signs yet, often that is not what a person wants to hear when they go for a regular check-up. Most people do not heed early warning signs. They only pay attention when late signs occur such as the need for a stent, heart bypass surgery or treatment for a stroke.

Many of the lifestyle changes required to grow older in a healthy way are described by patients as too radical. To this I respond, "Isn't having your chest cut open for heart bypass surgery radical?"

Eating healthy food and exercising daily is not radical – it is what we need to get this country back in shape!

More and more people are becoming overweight and obese, developing chronic disease and cancer and dying at a young age. This does not need to happen and much can be avoided by living a clean, anti-inflammatory lifestyle. Cherish your health and enjoy each day in optimal wellness!

- Dr. Sal

Do You Truly Care About Your Health?

While at the American College of Lifestyle Medicine conference, I listened to Dr. James Beckerman, a cardiologist from Oregon, talk about the health benefits of exercise. He started his presentation reminding the audience that we are all on a journey, a pilgrimage. He told us that he asks his patients, "Why do you want to be healthy?" He attempts to get to know his patients by understanding where they are on their health journey as well as understanding if and why they care about their health. In Dr. Beckerman's practice, he talks a lot about lifestyle behaviors, nutrition and exercise and even writes formal prescriptions for exercise. He showed a picture of a gentleman who intentionally went from being fit (like super fit!) to fat and then back to super fit again in order to prove the point that nature can be nurtured. Genes are not necessarily our destiny. We have much more influence over our genetics than we believe; and, when we decide to be fit and healthy, we can – it is all about the effort.

Dr. Beckerman talked about risk factors of heart disease and listed several along with the relative risk numbers. We know that a family history of premature heart disease before the age of fifty in a first-degree relative becomes a personal factor. Having this family history increases personal risk by about 24%. Other risks include the following: being overweight 33%, elevated cholesterol 45%, high blood sugar 63% and high blood pressure increases risk 67%, smoking increases the risk 89%. Those with a sedentary lifestyle, who are unfit, the risk of heart disease increases by 203%! This indicates that a person deemed unfit has twice the chance of developing heart disease, bringing a significant risk of premature death. These numbers highlight the value of exercise and the reason why most physicians talk with their patients about its benefits.

In relation to the word "formal," Dr. Beckerman spoke about the value of formal exercise versus just being active. He talked about a study done comparing individuals who sat most of the day but did a certain amount of formal, moderately intense exercise daily and compared this situation to someone who is active most of the day but does no formal exercise. The study found that the mostly sedentary person who exercises for 30 minutes per day has the same risk as an active person who does not exercise. The take-home message is: being active throughout the day is good yet, you should still schedule time for daily formal exercise. Formal exercise improves cardio respiratory fitness (CRF). This is what lowers our risk for heart disease and many other chronic illnesses.

The exercise evaluation Dr. Beckerman does with his patients includes having them keep a diary of how much they sit throughout the day and how much formal exercise they do. He wants them to be mindful of the amount of sitting because research shows that prolonged sitting is just as unhealthy as smoking cigarettes. He has them do a six-minute walking test, a good predictor of fitness and future health problems. He also measures what is called a Vo2 max. This is a formal measurement of the ability of the heart and lungs to get oxygen throughout the body. When the cells of the body are not supplied with proper amounts of blood, nutrients and oxygen, they are unable to function properly. Then, in time, the body begins to fail. Many wellness and fitness centers perform the Vo2 fitness test, however, if you are not able to have a formal Vo2 test done, you can go to the website www.worldfitnesslevel.org to do a calculation that is fairly close to the actual measured Vo2.

One interesting point he made was that people who receive a formal exercise prescription from their physician or health care provider actually do exercise more. I have seen this in my practice also. Dr. Beckerman talked about what is called the NTT (number to treat). This is the number of people that need to be treated with a certain therapy in order to create a benefit. Let's look at the NTT for statin use. Statin medications are used to lower cholesterol; the belief is that lowering a person's cholesterol will lower their risk of heart disease. The NTT for statins is 104.

When we look at the benefits of aspirin to lower the risk of heart disease, the number to treat is 1667; this is the number of people who need to take aspirin for one person to get the benefit. Next, when you look at the NTT for use of the Mediterranean diet to lower the risk of heart disease, the number is 61. Interestingly, this is lower than the number for statin use. This means that eating a Mediterranean diet appears to lower the risk of heart disease as much as using a statin medication. It is important to understand this occurs with people who do not already have heart or vascular disease. This is called primary prevention where health care works to prevent the problem from occurring in the first place. These numbers do not relate to folks who already have heart or vascular disease who probably need to be treated with, not only nutrition, exercise and a change in lifestyle, but possibly medications. When looking at the NTT for exercise, the number is 26 meaning that exercise has to be prescribed for 26 people in order for one person to increase their exercise. This number to treat is lower than other NTT numbers and highlights the value of a physician prescribing exercise. From these numbers, it is obvious many people must be treated to receive the intended benefit; nonetheless, this approach works. Think of the benefit a person would get in lowering the risk of heart disease if they exercise regularly, eats a healthy diet and when necessary, takes a statin medication to lower the cholesterol. The overall goal is to use all available therapies to become and stay healthy.

Thanks to progress in pharmaceutical science, we have many medications which improve lives. We have pills, procedures and surgeries that make a big difference in health care today yet, we have become a society too quick to reach for the pill or agree to a surgical procedure without knowing an alternative may be just as effective.

When someone is faced with an illness or a health problem, it is important to know all the available options. For example, if diet, exercise and weight reduction are able to achieve almost the same improvement in diabetic control, why would this not be the first option? There are no negative side effects of eating healthy food and regularly exercising. This is not the case with pills, procedures and surgery. Again, I emphasize -- when these methods of treatment are necessary, thank goodness they are available. The message is that often a change in lifestyle behavior is all that is needed.

Getting back to the question asked at the beginning of this article, "Do you truly care about your health and, if you do, what are you willing to do to care for, nourish and cherish it?" What are you willing to sacrifice to stay well? There is nothing more important than maintaining optimal health. This should be the first priority every day. Once you develop a healthy lifestyle action plan that becomes a part of your life, all else falls in line. Good health allows you to do everything that makes you happy and fulfilled.

- Dr. Sal

Healthy People, Healthy Planet

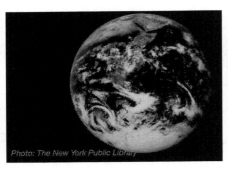

Photo: The New York Public Library

Recently I wrote an article about the U.S. dependence on oil for energy, the problems with global warming, national security and, of course, the health-care crisis. All of these issues fundamentally involve food one way or another. The production of food directly influences our dependence on oil. Agribusiness creates as much global warming as automobile fumes. The production of food also affects the security of the nation; many branches of the armed forces have found that recruits are not healthy. The health care crisis is directly related to food; the processing of food has dramatically altered the nutritional content of the standard American diet. Processed foods are the main reason for many of the chronic illnesses people in America suffer from daily. Food is the main cause, but also a significant part of the solution to the health care crisis.

Dr. Richard Oppenlander has written about how the production of food negatively influences the planet. He gives sobering statistics about the depletion of so many species of animals, insects and fish and how food production (especially meat and dairy) negatively impacts the environment. He makes a call to action for stopping the decline of the planet.

Currently, we are in the midst of a water shortage and in many cities and towns, a water drought. This is partially because we devote much of the nation's water supply to raising animals therefore, less water is available for human consumption. Currently, there are over seven billion people on the planet; this number will soon rise to nine billion. While we already produce enough food to feed everyone, much of the grain produced in the world goes to feeding animals. This is important since we still have many millions of people across the world suffering from starvation. We don't have time to waste. Our planet is suffering and the health of many people in the U.S. is declining rapidly. Each day more of our family members, friends, co-workers and neighbors develop chronic illness and cancer. Many die prematurely because of this.

216

Lifestyle medicine is making people aware of the natural things they can do to become and stay healthy including: eating truly healthy food, exercising daily, managing stress, getting enough sleep, loving others and being loved. It is well known that social support directly impacts a person's quality of life and longevity. When we look at places in the world where people live the longest, we see these simple elements are direct contributors to a good life. If you want to live a healthy life, you must have healthy lifestyle behaviors which promote and support optimal health.

Dr. Michael Greger is known as the king of evidence-based scientific information. Read his book, *How Not To Die*, and you will understand. Dr. Greger makes health recommendations only after he has thoroughly reviewed the science making sure the research is consistent. He is a firm believer of how plant-based nutrition improves chronic illness and, in many cases, prevents disease and cancer.

As many of the readers know, heart disease is the number-one killer in the U.S. and in most developed countries. Dr. Erkki Vartiainen, from Finland, has written about the Karelia project. It shows that a significant change in diet and lifestyle produces tremendous improvements in heart disease and mortality. By changing what the people of Karelia ate, they lowered the risk and incidence of heart disease by 80%!

A change in the way we live improves depression and anxiety which many people have today. The usual treatment is an anti-depressant medication. Since there are no medications without side effects, using an anti-depressant often creates side effects, adding to the primary problem. Weight gain is also common which may lead to depression. Lifestyle interventions, counselling and other support services should be part of the initial treatment protocol. Understanding the root cause of depression is instrumental in treatment and cure.

This **lifestyle medicine revolution** is something I am proud to be a part of and hope the readers will join me on the journey.

- Dr. Sal

DNA is Not Your Destiny ... Dinner Is!

" *DNA is not your destiny, dinner is!"* I have to thank Dr. Dean Ornish for this statement which means that genetics, our DNA, does not determine our destiny as much as our meals do. Dr. Amy Chappell, a neurologist from Naples, Florida, used Dr. Ornish's statement in a presentation she made on diabetes and Alzheimer's. The reason for using the statement was to explain that although a person might inherit bad genes, they might not get the intended disease depending on the lifestyle they live, especially in regard to what foods are eaten on a regular basis.

Dr. Chappell has talked about Alzheimer's as Type 3 Diabetes. She explains that excess sugar in the body negatively affects all organs, including the brain. She speaks of the ApoE gene that, when inherited, increases a person's risk for Alzheimer's. Yet, studies have shown that lifestyles either result in these bad genes being turned on or off, depending on lifestyle quality. In countries where inheritance of the ApoE gene is high and where the lifestyle is healthy, the incidence of the actual disease is low. This would seem to prove the statement: *DNA is not your destiny*. The second part of the statement, *dinner is*, certainly makes sense.

The production of food in recent years resulted in some of the most common sources of toxins that affect the function of our DNA. When we examine all processed foods (foods that come in a box or a bag) and even most animal products (red meat, chicken, pork, lunch meats and dairy), we find an overabundance of chemicals, hormones, bacteria and other non-food additives, none of which are nutritionally beneficial. As an example, for school presentations, I read the list of ingredients on a bag of Fruit Loops: Red 40, Turmeric extract color,

218

Yellow 6, Blue 1, Annatto extract color, and BHT for freshness. In the past I have read about these colorings and additives stating that there is research linking them to behavioral problems, allergies and other health problems in children. When the body has to deal with or metabolize chemicals that are not intended to be nutritional, often it does not know how to handle these foreign chemicals, creating allergies, autoimmune diseases and other chronic health problems. The result of this metabolic confusion might be the turning on of bad genes causing diseases such as Alzheimer's and other similarly devastating illnesses. In the last 100 years, we have seen the emergence of over 100 autoimmune diseases such as celiac, thyroiditis and different types of arthritis. Why have these illnesses developed? We must **look for the cause** and not just treat the symptoms.

Both Dr. Chappell and I have spoken about the generalities of Type 2 diabetes (aka adult-onset diabetes). My focus is mainly on how we can prevent, treat and reverse it -- the benefit of lifestyle in managing another disease thought to be inherited (diabetes). This is a disease caused more by lifestyle than DNA. Lifestyle will either create disease or create health, depending on how you live. The foundation for healthy living is on the dinner table!

Thousands of clinical studies have been done looking at food and its association to disease and health. The results of these studies are clear: the more processed foods a person eats, the more at risk they are for most chronic illnesses and common cancers people suffer from. When we choose to eat organic, non-processed, whole natural foods, we get less disease, live a better quality and longer life. Dr. Chappell and I both champion the CHIP program in our respective practices. This is the **Complete Health Improvement Program** (CHIP), a nine-week program that teaches the participants how to shop, cook and eat delicious, health promoting foods. This program helps people reverse many of their common health problems, enjoy more energy and good health than they have in years. The clinical results and the anecdotal reports are inspiring.

219

Dr. David Katz, from the American College of Lifestyle Medicine, has written: *health is delivered by our forks, feet and fingers.* When we use a fork to feed ourselves healthy food, use our feet to get regular exercise and don't use our fingers to smoke, we stay healthy and enjoy life! What you put on the plate determines your future health more than your DNA. To ensure a healthy life, fill your plate with fresh, whole, natural, unprocessed foods and enjoy a wonderful meal!

- Dr. Sal

Health Care Reform Starts With Me!

In Fort Myers, Florida, the *Lee Health* team members have been reaching out to other organizations across the nation to identify novel ways to integrate lifestyle behaviors into traditional medical care. Health care reform is not a governmental initiative but rather it is a grass roots effort starting with each individual interested in maintaining good health.

When individuals focus on health care, as opposed to sick care, positive things can happen. Our health care system is a sick care system. Often individuals wait for things to go wrong with their health (assuming that a lack of diagnosed disease is an indication of good health), then become involved to recapture good health. As most physicians and health care providers know, it is much more difficult to regain good health once it is lost. The YouTube video, ***Make Health Last***, is a very poignant view of how many in America spend the last few years of their lives in sickness, not wellness. This is in contrast to those places in the world where people live beyond 90 or even 100 years, a result of living a very healthy lifestyle.

The commonalities across five places in the world where people live longer than others include: healthy eating, regular physical activity, strong social support and a sense of purpose. Food is wholesome, natural and not processed. Activity includes daily walking and other functional behaviors not simply spending an hour a day on a treadmill going nowhere. The elderly in these places are revered and cared for their entire lives. As they age and become less functional, family and friends provide the physical and emotional support necessary to make aging graceful. These individuals continue

221

to maintain an active role in the family and community and a passion for living.

In recent years, many in the U.S. have attempted to fix the health (sick) care system but unfortunately, this has not been very successful. We continue to see more folks with chronic disease and cancer. The focus has been maintaining a system designed to cure rather than prevent disease. This is the reason I am passionate about spreading the message regarding the value of preventive health care. Developing an action plan for healthy living appears to be the solution to many of the health care problems people suffer from. To reform the health care system in America today, we must start reforming the way we live.

This healthy living action plan focuses on nutritious food. When we become mindful about eating healthy food, we provide our body with the essential nutrients to stay healthy and fight disease. When adding regular physical activity, we add to the benefits of eating healthy food. The addition of social support and a sense of purpose is important; and, if we are passionate about parts of our lives, the benefits are even greater!

In the event a health problem does occur, we need to ask the question, WHY? When a person is diagnosed with high blood pressure (hypertension), we must work diligently to find out why. Was it the result of a genetic/inherited disorder or the result of an unhealthy lifestyle, poor diet, lack of exercise, weight problem or possibly a medication side effect? Knowing the cause allows the patient and physician to develop a plan to treat the cause, not simply treat the symptom. This applies to other health problems such as high cholesterol, heartburn, chronic constipation and more. Getting to the root cause of the problem allows for the development of a treatment plan aimed to cure and prevent recurrence. Often, we see individuals having heart vessel bypass surgery going home after their surgery and get back to their pre-surgery unhealthy lifestyle. The individual is more prone to develop a recurrence since they did not deal with the cause. When a similar individual leaves the hospital armed with a healthy living action plan, they have less chance of returning with the same problem.

All this requires work; it is not easy to become and stay healthy. Everything in life that is valuable requires work and sacrifice. We have to be willing to do both, knowing that the benefits we gain far outweigh anything sacrificed to achieve optimal health.

Each day when you open your eyes and think about your priorities, recite these words:

> *"Health is my number one priority; without good health all other goals are less achievable. When I maintain optimal health, I can achieve all my goals and even help others achieve theirs. I bring value to others, my community and the world by guarding and nourishing my health. Health care reform starts with me!"*

- Dr. Sal

The Cure is in the Kitchen

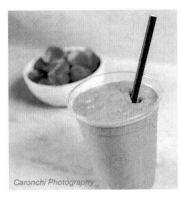
Caronchi Photography

The Cure is in the Kitchen is the title of an article I read in the *Experience Life* publication. The article described the Mayo Clinic teaching kitchen and how many of the physicians, health care providers and hospital administrators believe the cure to the health care crisis in America resides in the kitchen. I agree! Research shows that the majority of chronic illnesses and many common cancers occur as a result of an unhealthy lifestyle, with a major focus on unhealthy food. The standard America diet is disease promoting. Weight related medical problems include heart attacks, strokes, diabetes, even a greater risk for cancer.

In this article the author writes about a drug dealer who continues to live a dangerous life and has numerous visits to the emergency room for treatment of gunshot wounds. She makes an analogy to the persistence of an unhealthy lifestyle that many people lead even after being diagnosed with heart disease. Despite these diagnoses, they come into the emergency room multiple times with chest pain from angina (poor blood flow to the heart) which often is the result of a diet that continues to clog the arteries.

I have seen this scenario play out in real life in my medical practice hundreds of times. Even after having heart bypass surgery, many people return to their pre-surgery way of life and the disease continues to progress bringing them back to the emergency room.

The interesting statistics described in this article include many relating weight to chronic disease and cancer. One alarming statistic is that women who have survived   breast cancer and are significantly

224

overweight (BMI>30), have a 30% greater chance of recurrence and almost a 50% chance of dying from the cancer as a woman who has a normal weight (BMI< 25). According to the American Cancer Society, being overweight is related to 14% of cancer deaths in men and 20% in women, older than 50 years of age. More than 16% of strokes are associated with obesity and middle-aged men who are obese have a 60% greater chance of dying from a heart attack compared to a man with a healthy weight.

At the Mayo Clinic and many other health care institutions across the nation, health care providers are working to educate about the power of nutrition including nutrition along with other helpful therapies. Teaching kitchens are becoming the norm and this is part of the wellness plans at Lee Health. For several years many of the physicians, health care providers and hospital administrators have participated in a *Food is Medicine* committee developed to help educate health care providers regarding the value of nutrition in preventing disease. We have made tremendous gains organizing health care providers interested in helping people treat disease, also reversing and preventing disease.

One focus of this committee is to review the clinical research related to food and disease and contrast this with the evidence related to nutrition and health. Food in America is the standard American diet loaded with salt, sugar and fat – the three components of a meal destined to cause obesity, chronic illness and cancer. This is in contrast to a meal filled with unprocessed, whole, natural, delicious edibles. These foods sustain the body, provide low calorie energy, support the immune system and lead to a better quality of life and greater longevity. This explanation is necessary in order to understand the difference between food and nutrition.

The health of the nation and each individual living in it is dependent on what is on their breakfast, lunch and dinner plate. As the title states, *The Cure is in the Kitchen*, and this statement is so true! Whether it is your personal kitchen or the kitchen of a restaurant, what

225

you put on your plate will determine your present and future health. Nothing is more impactful on health than what you put on your fork. In addition, what you put on your feet also matters – your exercise sneakers; and, what you do not put in between your fingers — cigarettes. Exercise adds to the benefits of healthy nutrition, as do not smoking, minimizing stress and getting enough sleep. These are the foundations for a healthy living action plan.

Around 2500 years ago Hippocrates stated, "let food be thy medicine and medicine be thy food," and he could not have been more correct. A wonderful current day resource for nutrition education is Dr. Michael Greger's website, NutritionFacts.org. Many books have been written by national authorities on nutrition and healthy lifestyles including: Dr. Caldwell Esselstyn, Dr. T. Colin Campbell, Dr. Joel Fuhrman, Dr. David Katz, Dr. Garth Davis and Dr. Hans Diehl. One great way to learn how to cook healthy meals is to complete the online course called *Culinary Rx*. Once you learn the fundamentals of nutrition, you will learn how to reorganize your kitchen and cook healthy meals. The Culinary Rx program is one of many programs that will allow you to continue on your journey toward optimal health.

- Dr. Sal

Would a Preventative Approach be More Cost Effective?

An article in *The Wall Street Journal* reported that one pharmaceutical company spent $1 billion researching a medication thought to be useful in breaking down the plaques that appear to cause Alzheimer's disease; the results have been disappointing. I read this article twice to be sure I understood the contents since the $1 billion price tag seemed unbelievable — yet that is the correct amount!

When we look at the most common reasons for death and disability in the U.S., we learn more than five million people are living with Alzheimer's dementia (AD); and, the number is increasing annually. The financial toll pales in comparison to the physical and emotional toll this disease has on the individual and the family. Caregivers often have trouble as the affected individual is not aware of the total ramifications of the illness. The patient suffers a slow decline in memory and cognitive function, while the family deals with the loved one's inability to perform activities of daily living, activities which may become the responsibility of a caregiver. For the caregiver, this is a work schedule which takes a physical, mental and emotional toll.

With these facts, several questions come to mind including: would a preventive approach be more cost effective than doing research to cure or reverse disease? Would the results be more beneficial if additional money was spent on research defining the cause of the disease? Would the overall situation improve with the development of procedures and protocols aimed at prevention?

We know that the risk factors for AD include advanced age, educational level and a family history of neurodegenerative disease, head trauma as well as genetic predisposition. The latter involves

227

what is known as mutations/errors in the Apo E gene. When an abnormal gene develops, the individual has a higher likelihood of developing AD. These risk factors are very similar to the risk factors for cardiovascular disease (CVD). As mentioned, there is a genetic component involved in both AD and CVD yet many of the risk factors for both diseases have more to do with lifestyle than genetics.

The link between CVD and AD has been termed the heart-head connection and some autopsy studies have revealed that 80% of those who die with AD also had some degree of CVD. In this situation we use the term vascular dementia, as we know this is a total body blood flow problem leading to the development of CVD and AD. Essentially, this is poor circulation throughout the body.

The Apo E gene mutation is said to increase the risk of AD and CVD by about 25%. We know that not all people who inherit the abnormal gene develop the disease therefore, it appears other things control the occurrence of this illness. It is said that lifestyle behaviors can either turn on or turn off gene functions, meaning we might have more control over these bad genes than once believed. As such, genetics are not always our destiny.

When we look at the incidence of AD in the U.S. and compare it to the occurrence of AD in other countries, we see significant differences. Why is it that the disease occurs so commonly in the U.S. yet less often in other countries? The difference appears to be related to the lifestyle behaviors which certainly include what people eat and how active they are physically and mentally.

Prevention studies have been done including the DIAN study (the Dominantly Inherited Alzheimer's Network) which has been testing the usefulness of antibodies designed to decrease the accumulation of amyloid plaques in individuals with deterministic genes. These deterministic genes produce specific proteins in the brain which significantly increase the likelihood of developing AD. The goal of this study is to develop and use antibodies that rid the brain of these abnormal proteins as they develop in these high-risk individuals.

The A4 study (Anti Amyloid in Treatment of Asymptomatic Alzheimer's) was done with individuals 65-85 years of age, also looking to see if the amyloid plaque production could be delayed. Results from some of these studies have not been as encouraging as we would like, while there have been some positive animal studies. One study done with beagle dogs fed a diet high in antioxidants revealed improved memory and recall and, another study in mice reported improved learning, brain growth factors, vascular function and increased synapses (connections between nerve cells in the brain). In the latter study, they measured the level of BDNF (Brain Derived Neurotropic Factor) which has been described as a fertilizer for the brain. It appears that the simplest studies involving lifestyle behaviors (nutrition and exercise) have produced encouraging clinical results with minimal money invested.

For a person who asks, "what can I do to decrease my risk of getting AD (or CVD)?" the answer lies in a preventive health care strategy including: maintaining an ideal body weight, limiting alcohol, other brain toxins, avoiding cigarettes and other recreational drugs, exercising regularly, eating lots of vegetables, fruits and other foods high in antioxidants, staying socially connected and keeping the brain active by learning new things on a regular basis. If we want to decrease the risk of chronic illnesses, we must internalize healthy daily lifestyle behaviors and commit to maintaining this lifestyle. Research and anecdotal reports detail the positive effects of lifestyle on not only the quality of life but on longevity. Our focus should be on curing and reversing disease and working just as hard on preventing it!

- Dr. Sal

Lending a Helping Hand

A while ago I had the honor of participating in a charity event for Gigi's Playhouse, a worldwide network of Down's syndrome (DS) achievement centers. This network helps individuals with DS achieve all they can through free, result-driven programs for all ages, their families and communities. The charity event was a 10k (6.1 mile) race which started at 8 am. I was doing well until just before the one-mile mark when my foot hit a divot in the road, twisting my left ankle severely. I managed to stop myself from falling and finish the race with minimal pain however, that did not last long. Once the race ended, the pain increased. By the time I got home it was so severe I was unable to put weight on the ankle.

At this point you might be thinking — what does this have to do with the title of the story or to do with health? So, let me explain. First, Down's syndrome is a genetic disorder caused by the presence of all or part of a third copy of chromosome 21 (normally there are only two copies of each chromosome). DS typically is associated with physical growth delays, characteristic facial features and a wide range of intellectual abilities. I know about this health condition as much personally as professionally since my uncle, cousin and niece all have DS. From being around other DS adults and children for many years, I can tell you they are the most loving, gentle and kindhearted people you will ever meet. I actually began my career in medicine because of a beautiful DS boy I worked with in New York, named Andy.

Many people will call individuals with DS handicapped, disabled or other terms. I believe they have tremendous abilities enabling them to lend a helping hand. When you encounter a person with DS they immediately remind you of what is important in life:

kindness, gentleness, hugs and smiles. Initially, meeting a person with DS will brighten your mood and make your day better. Then, getting to know them will teach you about this genetic disorder that affects them physically and intellectually. Despite these conditions, individuals with DS do not let it affect them personally. This has taught me that a disability can often be overcome. It is the mental fortitude that allows a soldier returning from the war missing a limb or suffering from the effects of head trauma to achieve more than they could ever have imagined. Many times disabled people become more able-bodied (physically, mentally and emotionally) and end up helping themselves and others.

Personal injury or illness usually teaches us to become more sympathetic, empathetic and helpful to those suffering from either a genetically inherited disorder or an acquired illness. During the few days after my ankle injury, as I was hobbling around the house on crutches and understanding what life is like without full use of my legs, I thought more of how those with a similar but permanent disability deal with these challenges. You truly come to understand another when put in their shoes! This was a reminder to me to look for every opportunity to help others in need. Whether the individual is dealing with DS or loss of a limb, we all have the ability to lend a helping hand. When we do, we personally benefit from the help we give to others. Research has proven volunteerism benefits the one who gives as much as the one who receives.

From this I hope the reader learns and understands Down's Syndrome or other physical or intellectual challenges they may face. It is important, I feel, to internalize what it would be like to have any of these challenges and determine what might be done to make the life of another easier and happier. We are all on this earth to help one another. That is one of the goals for the thousands of professionals I have the pleasure of working with each day. Thank you for letting us be part of your health care.

- Dr. Sal

Exercise and Recovery Time

I f you have ever exercised and developed post exercise muscle soreness, you might have wondered if there was a way to quickly resolve the soreness before the next exercise session. I found a study published in the *Journal Nutrients* which looked at the effects of tart cherry juice on athletic performance and recovery time.

This United Kingdom research team conducted a double-blind, placebo-controlled study (meaning that neither the scientists performing the study nor those participating knew if they were getting the tart cherry juice or the placebo) and tested 16 semi-professional male soccer players randomly assigned to either the tart cherry juice arm of the study or the placebo control group. Participants drank one ounce of a commercially available tart cherry juice daily and the control group drank a calorie-matched fruit cordial. All participants were tested for athletic performance involving muscle strength tests as well as a 20-meter sprint. Across every performance measure, the individuals who drank the tart cherry juice performed better. Additionally, they had lower levels in their blood of a marker for inflammation, namely Interleukin-6 (IL-6). The athletes subjectively rated their muscle soreness. In the tart cherry juice group, the scores for soreness were lower in the 72 hours following the exercise testing.

Making time for exercise is certainly a great goal yet often individuals jump too quickly into a tough exercise routine. In a short period of time, they are feeling so sore and tired the exercise goes by the wayside. To avoid this scenario, a thoughtful plan should be developed to increase the chance of this new lifestyle behavior becoming a permanent part of daily life.

232

Energy is produced in every cell of the body by parts of the cell called the mitochondria. These internal organelles produce energy in the form of adenosine triphosphate (ATP). The process requires oxygen, glucose, healthy fatty acids, carnitine, vitamins and minerals. These macronutrients (fats and carbohydrates) and micronutrients (vitamins and minerals) are used in the chemical reactions ending up with the production of ATP. The cell then uses this energy to perform the various functions of the specific organ made up by these specialized cells. For example, if the cells are in the heart, the ATP makes the heart muscle cells contract so the heart is able to pump blood throughout the body. If the cells are in the brain, the ATP makes neurotransmitters, chemicals the cells in the brain use to communicate with one another. If the cells are in the skeletal muscles, the ATP makes amino acids, the building blocks for the proteins making up the skeletal muscles. If the cells are in the adrenal glands, the ATP makes the dozens of hormones the body and brain need to function and stay healthy.

In addition to providing the cells with the various macro and micro nutrients as mentioned, oxygen is needed. The lungs must be healthy to take in proper amounts of oxygen and the heart needs to be healthy to efficiently pump the oxygen filled blood to all the cells of the body. More information about cell energy and cell functions may be found at www.nature.com.

Poor nutrition, smoking and a lack of exercise impairs the cells' ability to make energy. An individual might complain of chronic fatigue, poor exercise tolerance and a limited ability to perform activities of daily life due to the following: not eating healthy food, getting the proper amounts of fats, carbohydrates, proteins, vitamin and minerals, smoking (impairing the function of the lungs), and exercising to keep the heart healthy. All these add up to a decreased ability of the cells to produce ATP energy.

Once the person creates the initial part of a healthy lifestyle, the cells are able to make proper amounts of ATP energy; they are ready to create an exercise routine. If you have not been regularly exercising, visit with your physician/health care provider to be sure you do not need a stress test first. Many people develop occult/hidden cardiovascular disease as they age which sometimes occurs without symptoms. Once you know your heart is healthy, work with an exercise specialist to develop an exercise routine. The routine should include aerobic exercise, weight lifting (or resistance machines), flexibility/stretching exercises, and core exercises to strengthen the abdominal muscles and back. The latter is very helpful to avoid back injuries. The stronger the back and abdominal muscles, the less the likelihood of developing back strains and sprains. The reader might find it helpful to work with a nutritionist knowledgeable in sports nutrition if they plan on any intense exercising.

After starting regular physical activity, you might try the tart cherry juice to see if it improves your exercise tolerance and recovery time. Exercise tolerance is a progression. As you continue exercising, your muscles, heart and lungs get stronger. Your body adjusts to the added stress improving the quality of life and, as clinical studies show, longevity.

In summary, mindful eating improves exercise tolerance while tart cherry juice may help with recovery time. Research also shows that regular exercise decreases the risk and incidence of chronic illnesses including: cardiovascular disease, diabetes, obesity, metabolic syndrome, dementia and more.

- Dr. Sal

Chronic Fatigue

Sleep deprivation is tolerable for a short period of time; when fatigue persists for weeks or even months, it may be a sign of a deeper health problem. It then becomes important to seek medical attention, get to the root cause of the problem and make a diagnosis. Many physical as well as psychological health conditions can cause chronic fatigue including: anemia, low thyroid, heart failure, chronic infections, cancers, hormone imbalance, adrenal fatigue, fibromyalgia, anxiety and depression.

Anemia is a condition where the body does not have enough red blood cells (RBCs). Red blood cells carry oxygen to all cells of the body. When there is a shortage of RBCs, all vital organs are affected and the individual complains of being chronically tired. In addition to oxygen, the RBCs carry other nutrients essential for good health. As such, the individual is chronically tired, and might also complain of mental fogginess, shortness of breath, chest pain associated with activity or, an inability to tolerate activity. Causes of anemia include blood loss, decreased production of RBCs or the destruction from various reasons. Blood can be lost from the intestines with colitis or a cancer. When a female suffers from heavy menstrual periods, she may become anemic. In cases where RBCs are not being produced properly or being destroyed, anemia develops. In all these situations, a comprehensive evaluation is required and might include a colonoscopy to look for bleeding in the large intestine, a bone marrow biopsy if there is suspicion that production or destruction of RBCs is the problem or blood tests looking for iron, B12 deficiency or other nutrient deficiency. Treatment depends on the reason found for the anemia which resolves the symptoms and corrects the underlying cause.

Low thyroid (hypothyroidism) is another reason for chronic fatigue. The thyroid gland is located in the front portion of the neck just above the sternum (chest bone). The main function is to regulate metabolism. When the thyroid hormone is not balanced, the body is unable to properly use carbohydrates, fats and proteins (macro nutrients). Hypothyroidism symptoms include: chronic fatigue, dryness of the skin, brittleness of the hair and nails, constipation, weight gain and an overall feeling of slowing down. The cause of hypothyroidism in many cases is autoimmune indicating the body is making antibodies against its own thyroid gland. Autoimmune thyroiditis, as it is called, can be caused by a viral illness yet in many situations, the cause is not identified. It is important to identify the reasons why the body's immune system is not working properly and treat the cause. In most of these situations the individual requires prescription thyroid hormone pills which resolves the hormone imbalance.

Heart failure is another condition which causes chronic fatigue. This occurs because the heart is unable to pump the proper amount of blood. The heart then is unable to deliver oxygen and nutrients required to the body and the brain. Symptoms are similar to those for anemia. The most common reasons for heart failure include chronically elevated blood pressure (hypertension) and heart attacks. The latter occurs because of poor circulation to the heart (arteriosclerosis/hardening of the arteries). When a heart attack damages the main pumping chamber of the heart (the left ventricle), the heart becomes weak and flabby leading to congestive heart failure. Blood and other fluids accumulate in the lungs making oxygen transfer from the lungs into the red blood cells difficult. If the proper amount of oxygen is not transported into the red blood cells, the individual suffers many symptoms, including chronic fatigue. Treatments for high blood pressure and elevated cholesterol are essential to strengthen the pumping function of the heart.

Chronic fatigue may also result from chronic infections causing persistent inflammation in the body. The ongoing infection uses up critical nutrients and the individual eventually becomes nutrient depleted. As the body attempts to clear the infection, systemic (overall) inflammation stresses the body and the individual complains of unending fatigue. Blood tests and cultures for viruses, bacteria and fungal infections are performed to make a diagnosis. Treatment depends on the basis for the infection. The situation can be similar for those individuals who have occult/hidden cancers. As a cancer starts to grow, it initially causes minimal symptoms which might be described benignly as *"I'm just tired."* If it continues to grow, the individual experiences more symptoms and definite signs of cancer develop. This is why visiting a physician or health care provider is so important. If a person starts feeling tired despite trying to get more sleep or eating better and the fatigue continues, they should see a doctor as soon as possible. At this point, a complete examination is important after the physician takes a complete history and then decides on the necessary tests needed to make a diagnosis.

Many hormone imbalances can be associated with chronic fatigue, especially the adrenal hormones, cortisol and DHEA. Cortisol is the stress hormone and when an acute stressful event occurs, the cortisol level rises and the individual is able to deal with the acute stress. This is the fight or flight response. When the stress is persistent over long periods of time, the cortisol response begins to fail. The person experiences what is termed adrenal fatigue. The adrenal glands are no longer able to keep up with the demand; cortisol and DHEA levels begin to fall. When this occurs, the individual is less able to metabolize nutrients and may develop periods of low-blood sugar. Blood pressure can be affected as fluid and electrolyte imbalances occur. Imbalances may also occur with hormones affecting libido, mental clarity and overall energy. One of the best ways to diagnose adrenal fatigue is by measuring the levels of cortisol in a saliva sample taken upon getting out of bed, at noon, 5 pm and then at bedtime.

Fibromyalgia is a common diagnosis made when individuals suffer from chronic, diffuse muscle soreness, generalize weakness and chronic fatigue. As these symptoms occur frequently and persistently, many individuals with fibromyalgia suffer from chronic anxiety and/or depression. Traditional therapies for both anxiety and depression can sometimes exacerbate the fatigue associated with fibromyalgia since anti-anxiety and anti-depressant medications may cause fatigue. Fibromyalgia, like many other chronic illnesses, is associated with systemic inflammation. This means the body is inflamed. The goal is to identify the root cause of the inflammation and treat the cause, not just the symptom. There are many causes of systemic inflammation including thousands of added chemicals in the foods we eat, water we drink and in all the products we use in daily life such as cleaning supplies, cosmetics or deodorants. Even the air we breathe can be toxic depending on where a person lives. Trying to live as clean a life as possible is one great way to decreases systemic inflammation.

In summary, fatigue might simply be the result of sleep deprivation. If it persists, it is most important to seek medical attention. Information for this article was taken from *Harrison's Principles of Internal Medicine* and from Dr. James Wilson's book on *Adrenal Fatigue*.

- Dr. Sal

The Importance of a Strong Immune System

Over the past several decades, clinical evidence has revealed an increasing incidence of allergies, asthma and autoimmune diseases. These are all illnesses where the body makes antibodies which actually attack itself. Medical professionals continue to diagnose and treat conditions such as allergic upper respiratory illnesses, allergic dermatitis (inflammation of the skin), multiple sclerosis (MS), type 1 diabetes (which usually starts in early life), inflammatory bowel diseases such as Crohn's disease and hay fever.

At the same time, in many developed countries, there has been an obvious decrease in the incidence of many infectious diseases as a result of the use of antibiotics, vaccines and improvements in hygiene. From 1950-2000 in the U.S. there was a tremendous decline in the incidence of tuberculosis, rheumatic fever, measles, mumps and hepatitis A.

As a result of the above statements, questions arise. Are naturally acquired infections helpful? Are prescription antibiotics used to fight infections harmful to the immune system? These are important questions about knowing how to bolster the functions of the immune system.

One interesting fact regarding allergic and autoimmune diseases is that, for certain diseases, there is a north-south gradient, meaning that the incidence of this disease changes as one moves from north to south. This scenario is true in the U.S. for MS and there is some evidence this is also true for type 1 diabetes. In Europe, allergies and Crohn's disease show a north–south gradient; in Australia, similar differences are seen in relation to MS.

Genetics seem to play a role in these differences, while the environmental effects on genetics seem to be even more crucial. This appears to be evident when individuals migrate from one country to another, going from an area of low to high incidence of a particular disease. If genetics alone was the primary factor in the development of the disease, individuals would develop the disease regardless of where they were living. If genetics predisposes an individual to an illness and environmental factors play a role in turning on bad genes, moving to an area where environmental factors are present would result in expression of the disease meaning the person develops the illness when he moves to a new country. This appears to be true for MS, type 1 diabetes and asthma.

These differences are also seen with the Lupus disease where the incidence is lower in western Africans (those living in their native country) as compared to black Americans (immigrants). Both populations are from the same ethnic group yet, the environment in which they live seems to bring out the susceptibility to the disease.

In addition to where a person lives, it appears that the socioeconomic status influences the occurrence of autoimmune illnesses such as type 1 diabetes, MS and Crohn's colitis. The explanation for this appears to be a more developed immune system as a result of increased exposure to infections. The latter occurs in lower socio-economic conditions because of more water contamination, poorer housing conditions and increased exposure to other individuals with infections. It appears that exposure to infections boosts the immune system keeping it regulated, therefore, these individuals are less susceptible to autoimmune illnesses.

A similar situation arises in children who attend day care. The earlier a child is in daycare and the higher the number of infections, the lower the incidence of autoimmune illnesses. Again, exposure to infections in early life appears to prime the immune system and influence its normal function. Children with older siblings also seem to have protection against autoimmune diseases. Situations which stress the immune system appear to be helpful.

This situation is different when it comes to the microbiome, the environment in the GI tract where millions of bacteria live and influence our health and/or susceptibility to disease. The microbiome starts to develop when a child is born and when the child is born vaginally, normal/helpful bacteria from the mother are passed to the child and live in the GI tract. The bacteria which make up the microbiome perform many healthful functions for the individual. When the child receives a dose of an antibiotic, the microbiome is disrupted and over time this may affect the child's susceptibility to autoimmune illnesses. The administration of antibiotics to children has been suspected to increase the risk of asthma and allergies. Researchers have observed the use of antibiotics in the first year of life increased the risk of asthma or other allergic diseases in children with a genetic predisposition. C-section deliveries also appear to increase the risk of autoimmune illnesses. In this situation, the child bypasses the normal path which allows them to be inoculated with the mother's normal bacteria. The child's microbiome becomes initially populated with bacteria from the mother's skin (different bacteria from the mother's vagina). Thus, the child's immune system develops differently. There is also some evidence to suggest that exposure of the mother to viral infections before the child is born influences the child's risk of developing an autoimmune illness later in life. As with other parts of the body, the child's immune system is also developing while they are in the womb.

Other factors that may influence the rate of allergies and autoimmune diseases include climate, air pollution and certainly diet. The latter is most interesting since the composition of food products in the last 100 years has changed dramatically. The nutritional content has decreased, and the number of contaminants has increased. Research has shown that foods in the standard American diet contain many hundreds of harmful chemicals, pesticides, antibiotics,

241

hormones, fecal bacteria and viruses. Vitamin D deficiency also appears to increase the risk of type 1 diabetes and multiple sclerosis.

So, the questions continue to arise: are naturally acquired infections helpful or harmful and do they protect us from developing autoimmune illnesses such as type 1 diabetes, asthma, allergies and MS? Are vaccinations helpful or do they negatively influence the function of the immune system relating to autoimmune illnesses? In regard to the latter, the research is inconclusive. It is important to stress that there are no solid data indicating either a positive or a negative role of vaccinations in the development of autoimmune or allergic diseases. The potential benefit of antibiotic therapy in situations in which the pathogenic role of a bacterium is doubtful should be carefully assessed. When a bacterial infection is not a certainty, the use of an antibiotic is probably more harmful than helpful since, as explained above, it negatively affects the microbiome. In addition to killing the helpful bacteria living in the gut, this situation allows for the growth of pathogenic (harmful) bacteria in the gut that may become resistant to commonly used antibiotics.

The immune system starts to develop in utero before the child is even born. The health of the mother influences the development of the child's immune system as does the method of delivery (normal vaginal birth versus C-section). The early use of antibiotics, as well as the child's exposure to infections affects the normal development and lifetime function of the immune system. When the immune system becomes hyperactive, autoimmune diseases may develop as the body now produces antibodies to itself. There is a delicate balance between the normal function of the immune system (so that it helps fight infections) and the development of auto antibodies (possibly resulting in the development of diabetes, MS, and thyroid disease). Important things to keep the immune system functioning normally include: eating healthy foods, decreasing overall stress, limiting exposure to chemicals/other toxins and in some cases taking extra vitamins and supplements to boost the immune system.

Much of the research for this article was obtained from *Harrison's Principles of Internal Medicine* and various national infectious disease journals.

- Dr. Sal

Lee Health Is Committed to Prevention

As Lee Health's system medical director of wellness and employee health, one of my major roles is educating employees, dependents and our community neighbors on how to become and stay healthy. For several years I have had the honor of working with dozens of professionals within Lee Health and Lee County, Florida on many projects to achieve these goals.

Since 2010 we have been blessed by the educational lectures from national authorities on health and wellness including: Dr. T. Colin Campbell, author of *The China Study*, Hans Diehl from the *CHIP* program, Dr. Phil Tuso from Kaiser Permanente, triathlete Brendan Brazier, Dr. Joel Fuhrman, author of *Eat to Live* and *The End of Heart Disease*, Dr. Michael Greger, author of *How Not to Die*, Dr. Marc Braman from the American College of Lifestyle Medicine, Dr. Caldwell Esselstyn, author of *Reversing Heart Disease* and Nelson Campbell from PlantPure Nation. Dr. Erkki Vartiainen talked on experiences from the North Karelia Project in Finland.

The Complete Health Improvement Program (CHIP), founded by Hans Diehl, is a plant-based nutrition program we have used with hundreds of Lee Health employees, spouses and many community folks since 2010. CHIP facilitator, Kathy Reynaert, has been instrumental in this nine-week program that has helped individuals achieve tremendous improvements in blood pressure, cholesterol levels, weight and diabetes levels.

We have also had lectures delivered by several local physician authorities on wellness including: Dr. Brian Taschner (Cardiologist), Dr. Jose Colon (Neurologist & Sleep specialist), Dr. Sebastian Klisiewicz (Physical Medicine and Rehabilitation specialist), Dr.

Heather Auld (Integrative Medicine) and Dr. Teresa Spano (Naturopathic consultant). They volunteer their time by speaking to public and professional audiences regarding the value of healthy eating and healthy lifestyle behaviors such as sleep, stress management and other methods of staying well in addition to pharmaceuticals.

The 5-2-1-0 nutrition collaborative is a healthy behavior change program which we used with over 300 children in the Lee Health day care centers. This program encourages and teaches young individuals ages 3-4 years to focus on eating 5 servings of vegetables and fruits daily; limiting screen time (TV, computers, etc.) to no more than 2 hours per day; making sure to get at least 1 hour of physical activity daily and to have 0 sugary drinks daily. This successful program is helping children establish healthy behaviors and will guide them in their formative years. I believe this concept should be adopted by people of all ages.

The Lee Health food and nutrition team completed a multi-year malnutrition study that identified many hospitalized individuals who were malnourished at the time of admission and provided them with an innovative solution for inpatient medical care. It also provided them with an after-discharge four-week supply of therapeutically appropriate meals. This extended care program has resulted in improved health outcomes plus significantly reduced readmission rates. This program called *Flavor Harvest @ Home* has been recognized nationally as an innovative nutrition solution supporting the concept of healing at home. By simply making sure individuals have healthy food to eat upon discharge, their medical conditions improved, and they were less often readmitted.

Lee Health conducted a whole food, plant-based nutrition research project with over 200 employees. This healthy nutrition program is a natural solution designed to help improve blood pressure, high cholesterol levels, weight related medical problems and more. These individuals ate a plant-based diet for 60 days, completed blood pressure and lab tests before and at the end. In a similar program run through Employee Health, most of the participants find significant subjective improvements in energy level, cognitive function and overall wellness.

Nutritionists/Dietitians are now in several of the Lee Physician Group (LPG) offices offering personalized nutritional consultations and guidance to patients in need and have been invaluable in helping design action plans for patients to improve their health through better nutrition.

Lee Health is concerned with the health of its patients and also the health of its employees and leaders. As system medical director of employee health, I work with Advanced Nurse Practitioners (ARNPs) who visit on average with 17,000 employees and spouses a year helping them with acute medical problems and their wellness goals. Several Lee Health executives have completed a wellness pilot program that enabled them to improve health risks as they modeled healthy lifestyle behaviors showing their commitment to health and wellness. They emphasized the importance of walking the walk and talking the talk when it comes to healthy living.

Lee Health's food and nutrition team has done a fabulous job of creating healthy meals for employees and the public at hospital cafés. Under the direction of Larry Altier, the chefs have been showcasing healthy, plant-based foods, knowing that health care starts with the food a person eats on a daily basis. Their innovative concept called VeggieFare provides Lee Health employees with over two dozen different whole food options daily in a made-to-order format. From this endeavor we have created a wide assortment of healthy grab-and-go meals for those pressed for time.

Christin Collins, Lee Health's liaison with community leaders, has been a champion of lifestyle medicine. The goal is to help create awareness of the importance of striving for optimal health and a sense of community among participants.

Since 2010, I have been working with almost 100 health care professionals (physicians, nurses, nurse practitioners, dietitians and hospital administrators) about using food as medicine. We call this committee Food is Medicine (FIM). With an intentional focus on helping physicians and patients understand the value of food as medicine, we have shown the medical community that healthy food often is just as effective as prescription medicines and other traditional therapies to decrease health risks and control chronic illnesses such as heart disease, diabetes and obesity. We emphasize that healthy food needs to be added to traditional medical practices to give each individual the best chance to attain optimal health.

At the Cape Coral Hospital campus of Lee Health, leadership has been instrumental in designing an Optimal Healing Environment, a place where patients and families can have the best chance of achieving optimal health. The word optimal is underscored since the goal is to be optimally well, not simply to be without disease.

The Healthy Life Center in Estero opened in December 2015. The first-of-its-kind health information and education center provides a variety of services and education that support healthy lifestyles, early detection of disease and chronic disease management. Along with connecting visitors to health screening programs, lectures, clinical programs and services, the staff of personal health advocates and schedulers link patients to physicians, health care specialists, outpatient services and community partners. In its first year of operation, more than 7,500 people visited the Center attending over 400 activities such as cooking demonstrations, lectures on healthy aging, brain health, integrative medicine, healthy hearts and joints, sleep and technology to keep healthy.

The Lee Health Solutions department focuses on educating people living with chronic diseases, and those who want to live a healthier life. The diabetes self-management program has been successful in helping participants improve their blood sugar control and reduce the risk of complications from diabetes. In addition, this department offers outpatient dietician counseling to help participants lose weight. They also provide guidance for those needing specialized nutrition plans based on their chronic health conditions. Free community programs are held for chronic pain and disease management. One of the goals for those who work in this department is to help individuals understand and take an active role in improving their health.

Personally, one of the most exciting parts of my job is writing articles and giving public presentations on health and wellness. It is exciting to work with people who truly want to become and stay healthy. In the Employee Health clinic, I have worked with hundreds of people on weight management and other health risk factors who are pleased with their success. These folks prove that adoption of healthy lifestyle behaviors each day does as much to improve health as traditional medical therapies.

Lee Memorial Health System transitioned into a new and improved Lee Health, the 16,000+ employees, physicians and volunteers continue to focus on treating acute and chronic illnesses and on helping people become and stay healthy. The goal is to keep people well and out of the hospital. By avoiding illness and disease we can create a community of healthy, fit, vibrant, productive individuals as well as lower health care costs, improve the overall quality of life for each individual and the community.

- Dr. Sal

Should You Take a Multivitamin?

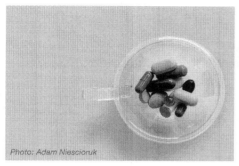
Photo: Adam Niescioruk

What is the clinical evidence regarding the usefulness of multivitamins? Much is written about the health benefits and much of this is anecdotal; therefore, we must look at the clinical evidence. Cardiovascular disease (CVD) and cancer are the number one and two causes of death in developed countries. A Harvard study in 2012 involving male physicians found an 8% decreased risk of cancer among those taking a multivitamin over 11 years. There was no beneficial effect on heart attacks or strokes.

Two clinical trials reported in the 2013 edition of the *Annals of Internal Medicine* found that multivitamins did not reduce the risk of age-related cognitive decline or heart attacks. In 2014, the US Preventive Services Task Force (USPSTF) looked at 25 clinical trials on vitamin/supplement use and determined there was not enough evidence to determine the benefits and harms associated with the use of multivitamins. It is obvious that the clinical evidence was conflicting and confusing. We can glean more useful information if we look at specific supplements as opposed to the use of a typical multivitamin.

Recently I wrote about the health benefits of turmeric, the spice that comes from the *curcuma longa* plant. Clinical evidence shows benefits in cardiovascular disease, insulin sensitivity, arthritis pain and even in ulcerative colitis. Glucosamine and chondroitin are other commonly used supplements for arthritic pain. Multiple clinical trials have been done in various countries and almost all report no

249

significant benefit as compared to a placebo. The Berkley School of
Public Health, *Wellness Report*, details seven clinical trials in which all
but one appear to be consistent. In my clinical practice, most patients
taking glucosamine and chondroitin do report a decrease in arthritic
pain and therefore, this might represent a placebo effect — simply by
taking a pill makes a person feel better. The side effects of
glucosamine are minimal. Some people with shellfish allergies may
have a problem since glucosamine is made from the shells of
shellfish. Chondroitin is made from the cartilage of cows and pigs;
there have been some reports of problems in those taking blood
thinners.

Next, let's consider the benefits of antioxidant supplements.
Oxidation within the body is sometimes explained as rusting of the
cells from within. The chemical reactions occurring inside all cells
produce reactive oxygen species (ROS), the small particles that cause
the oxidation/rusting. Obviously, this is not healthy for the cells
hence, the body produces antioxidants to relieve this stress. What does
the clinical evidence show regarding the use of antioxidant
supplements? Exercise is a stress to the body and when a person
exercises, they produce more oxidative stress (more of these ROS).
One clinical trial in Germany in 2009 done with high doses of
antioxidants did not show any improvement in insulin sensitivity.

Another study reported in the *Journal of Physiology* in 2014
reported benefits regarding the cellular adaptations to exercise (the
creation of new muscle mitochondria that make energy for the cells,
muscle growth in response to exercise and improvements in insulin
sensitivity). In looking at the studies to decide if taking antioxidants is
truly useful, it is difficult to decide since the answer depends on the
type and amount of the antioxidant used, how long they are taken, the
age and fitness of the person using them and even the type of exercise
they are doing. There are ways to measure the antioxidant levels in the
body (a skin method and a blood test method). These tests help the
physician and the patient decide if antioxidant supplement use may be

helpful. Eating lots of vegetables and a few fruits daily is a simple solution; because this provides you with antioxidants, fiber, vitamins, minerals and other chemicals truly known to keep a person healthy.

In relation to exercise, many people take supplements advertised to boost energy. Most of these supplements or energy drinks contain unhealthy levels of sugar and caffeine. High levels of sugar significantly increase a person's risk of not only diabetes, but also cardiovascular disease, dementia, obesity and premature aging. High levels of caffeine can irritate the heart, cause palpitations and irregular heart beating. Other supplements used by avid exercisers include creatine and amino acids. Creatine is made up of three amino acids (building blocks for proteins) and is involved in the production of ATP (energy for the cells). A 2010 review of creatine reported in the International Society of Sports Nutrition concluded that creatine is an effective supplement to boost muscle mass and strength to increase the capacity for high intensity exercise such as sprinting, jumping and weight lifting. Amino acid supplements are also used by avid exercisers, as are protein supplements, but often are used in excessive amounts. The recommended amount of protein per day is generally around one gram per kilogram of weight (70 grams for a normal weight male). If a person is doing heavy exercise on a regular basis, they may need more protein in the diet; while in excess, there is a concern for kidney function. I would refer individuals to a sports nutritionist if interested in taking protein, creatine or amino acid supplements as a way to build muscle. In most cases, eating healthy sources of protein (vegetables, quinoa, seeds, beans and grass-fed meats) supplies the needed amount of amino acids and protein to build and maintain healthy muscles.

One way to determine if a person is getting the proper amounts of vitamins, minerals, antioxidants and other helpful chemicals, is to perform a blood micronutrient test (MNT). This is a comprehensive analysis of all the vitamins, minerals and antioxidants reporting any deficiencies. With this information, the physician/health care provider

251

and the patient can then make an action plan which should focus on improving the diet. This is the best way to take in the necessary micronutrients. Once this is done and the individual eats the new and improved diet for several months, the MNT can be repeated to determine the effects. If deficiencies still persist then supplements may be added to the food portion of the nutrition plan. In many cases, tweaking the diet alone brings the levels of vitamins, minerals and antioxidants up to an optimal, healthy level.

In summary, vitamins and other supplements may be helpful to optimize health, yet there is nothing better than eating healthy foods to achieve this goal. A good guideline is eating at least six servings of vegetables daily, one to two servings of fruits, proper amounts of healthy protein as detailed above, and drinking six to eight glasses of water daily. Moderately intense exercise 30 minutes a day is important and minimizing stress by getting at least seven hours of quality sleep at night. This is a great healthy living action plan!

- Dr. Sal

February is Heart Health

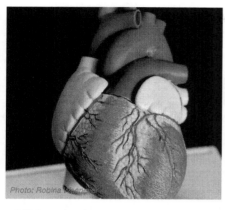

Photo: Robina

Heart disease is the number one killer in the U.S. and most developed countries; and, significantly preventable! Cardiovascular disease (CVD) in many cases occurs more as a result of lifestyle than genetics.

Often when a person has a family history of CVD, it is more apt to be related to everyone in the family living the same unhealthy lifestyle, as opposed to a true genetic susceptibility to the disease. In addition to a family history of premature heart disease as a risk factor, other risk factors include: smoking, high total and LDL (bad) cholesterol, low HDL (good) cholesterol, the presence of diabetes, high systolic blood pressure and obesity. What is important about these risk factors is that most, if not all, are controllable in distinction to the other risk factors: age, race and gender. Certainly, it can be argued that diabetes is less of a controllable risk factor since it appears this disease has some genetic susceptibility. Since the onset of diabetes is significantly related to obesity and lifestyle, it appears we have more control over the development of diabetes than previously thought. What supports this statement is the fact that the majority of diabetes cases (actually over 90%) occur in adulthood and are related to obesity, insulin resistance and an unhealthy lifestyle. Another sobering concern is that this so-called disease of adulthood is now being diagnosed in younger adolescents and children. In most situations, this is related to the individual being overweight while

253

eating more of the standard America diet – high in sugar, salt and saturated fat.

When we examine the reason CVD develops, it appears to be the result of multiple metabolic problems; this is one reason we are now using the term cardio-metabolic disease as opposed to heart disease or CVD. According to the University of California, Berkley School of Public Health *Wellness Report* from 2017, plaque formation begins with LDL cholesterol getting into the walls of the arteries causing inflammation. The operative word here is inflammation, since this appears to be the root cause of several diseases including heart and other vascular diseases such as vascular dementia and strokes. This report also discussed the damage to the arterial walls caused by high blood pressure and cigarette smoke and we must also include high blood sugar. Diabetes is considered a cardiovascular equivalent, meaning that a person with diabetes has the same risk of having a heart attack or a stroke as a person already diagnosed with CVD.

According to the Berkley report, scientists first identified the link between elevated cholesterol and heart disease in the early 1900s. The importance of high cholesterol in CVD became more evident in 1948, when data was collected from the on-going *Framingham Heart Study*. Over the last 50-60 years the importance of lowering LDL cholesterol has solidified as one way to significantly decrease the risk and incidence of CVD. With this information, the next question to answer is: what is the best way to lower cholesterol to decrease the risk of having a heart attack or a stroke? Fortunately, the answer includes multiple ways. As per the ACC/AHA guidelines, many individuals may benefit by taking a statin medication. Additional benefit is achieved with the addition of lifestyle modification such as a diet which includes healthy fats (flax, walnuts, salmon and avocado) and minimizing processed foods to lower the intake of simple sugars and excess salt. Regular physical activity, stress management, social support and quality sleep also help lower blood pressure and decrease inflammation throughout the body.

Calculating the 10-year risk of developing heart disease is helpful for all. The risk calculator at www.cvriskcalculator.com takes into account the age, gender, race, total and HDL cholesterol, systolic blood pressure, the presence of diabetes, if you smoke or are on high blood pressure medication. I recommend everyone access this website, calculate their score and discuss it with their physician/health care provider.

In addition to the above risk factors, the physician makes a full assessment of risk for CVD, they will ask about the presence of symptoms such as chest pain or shortness of breath with exertion, palpitations, lightheadedness or dizziness with activity. Once all this information is available, it is imperative to develop a healthy living action plan. This can be done in conjunction with a physician, a nutritionist/dietician, an exercise specialist and wellness coach. Once an action plan is in place for a certain time period, success can be assessed by re-measuring the lipid levels, blood glucose levels, blood pressure, weight and BMI. In my clinic I find it helpful to work with my patients on a wellness action plan so the person becomes and stays healthy. The goal of staying healthy cannot be overstated. Each day we are all aging yet CVD is not a disease of aging. In most cases it is a disease representing an unhealthy lifestyle and can be prevented. The goal is to assess risks for cardio-metabolic disease, understand risk factors, calculate risk score and develop an action plan that will decrease the risks and improve health. As a physician, it is very rewarding to help someone become and stay healthy; the individual becomes a role model for healthy living and will tell others. The wellness way of living spreads far and wide!

- Dr. Sal

How Not To Die

If you haven't read Dr. Michael Greger's book, *How Not to Die*, please do so! His book is filled with thousands of clinical references and recommendations on how to stay healthy and live a long, enjoyable life. When it comes to health, the goal is to stay healthy as one grows older, maintaining a high level of physical and intellectual function. People often say that health is the absence of disease yet this definition is limited. If you do not have a disease yet are not fully functional, you are not optimally healthy.

Dr. Greger's book is written in chapters dedicated to one body system at a time. He writes how not to die from heart disease, lung problems and immune dysfunction. His focus is on the cause of an illness and helps the reader to understand the risk factors. Dr. Greger's goal is decreasing these risk factors to avoid getting disease in the first place.

Heart disease is the number one killer in America today. It is important to look at what the clinical evidence regarding the development of what is better termed cardiovascular disease, but more specifically, cardio-metabolic disease. CVD/cardiovascular diseases include: heart attacks, strokes, high blood pressure and high cholesterol, vascular insufficiency in the legs, even erectile dysfunction and dementia. When blood flow to any organ is not optimal, illness occurs. Blood flow problems develop as a result of elevated LDL (bad cholesterol) which, when oxidized enters the inner walls of the arteries causing inflammation. A series of chemical reactions occur resulting in arteriosclerosis (hardening of the arteries). This creates high blood pressure and reduced blood flow. Plaque develops in the arteries; if the plaque occludes the artery, or a piece of the plaque breaks loose, blood flow downstream is significantly diminished — the individual has either a heart attack or a stroke. The clinical evidence shows that heart disease starts very early. In America, lifestyle has a significant impact on the development of many illnesses, including all the cardiovascular diseases mentioned. The term cardio-metabolic disease includes the metabolic changes that occur as a result of high fats in the blood, high blood sugar (which often is also found in a person with high cholesterol) and being overweight.

One chapter that is missing from Dr. Greger's book is: *How not to die from obesity*. Hundreds, if not thousands, of clinical research studies have proven the significant health consequences of obesity. In America, the obesity rate is over 30% for adults and the number continues to rise for adolescents and younger children. It is very unfortunate to see children now being diagnosed with type 2 diabetes, which has always been a disease of adults. This is the result of obesity, the standard America diet and the sedentary lifestyles that so many live today.

The second most common cause of death in the U.S. is cancer. There is a chapter, *How not to die from breast cancer* and others on prostate cancer and blood-born cancers. Each chapter details the risk factors and explains how a change in lifestyle positively affects these cancers by lowering the associated risks. One interesting point in the chapter on breast cancer is the association with melatonin (the so-called sleep hormone) production. A study published in the *International Archives of Occupational & Environmental Health* in 2015 reported on the increased incidence of breast cancer in women. Melatonin production was lower for night workers or those who do not sleep well. Melatonin is thought to play a role in suppression of cancer cells. Researchers from Brigham and Women's Hospital in Boston found that blind women have half the odds of breast cancer as sighted women; because they essentially live in darkness, their melatonin production is higher. This chapter in *How Not To Die* also

257

reviews the details of why inadequate fiber in the diet may increase the risk of breast cancer (European Journal of Nutrition, 2013). A report in the Journal of the National Cancer Institute from 2013 stated that every 20 grams of fiber intake was associated with a 15% lower risk of breast cancer. From these studies, it is helpful to know that improving sleep and increasing fiber in the diet may lower a women's risk of breast cancer.

The chapter on prostate cancer details the different rates of prostate cancer around the world. African Americans have a 30 times greater rate of prostate cancer as compared to Japanese men and a 120 times greater rate over Chinese men. A study in the Journal Prostate 1997 explains this might be due to the higher intake of animal protein and fat in the African men. One apparent protective factor in the diet of the Asian men is thought to be soy. This information is detailed as a meta-analysis in the *Journal BJU International* 2014. A meta-analysis is a review of many different research studies.

One interesting question posed in Dr. Greger's book is: why do centenarians (people who live beyond 100 years of age) seem to escape cancer? The answer seems to be related to the level of a growth hormone substance called IgF-1. The section in chapter 13 explains that the function of IgF-1 is to stimulate the development and growth of cells. As we age, the levels of IgF-1 normally decline since we do not need to produce as many cells. Certain individuals with higher than normal IgF-1 appear to have a higher risk of cancer, including prostate cancer. One factor associated with higher levels of IgF-1 is animal protein. Chapter 13 explains how limiting meat, eggs and dairy lowers the level of IgF-1 and decreases the risk of cancer (see reference in *Evidence Based Complement Alternative Medicine* 2011).

What is so enlightening to me about Dr. Greger's book is the clinical references and how he supports his statements with research studies done by a wide variety of authors across academic, private and public research sectors. When making recommendations on how to stay healthy, we must rely on valid, scientific and clinical evidence. Health recommendations should not be about one's opinion on what to do. In Dr. Greger's book, there are thousands of references supporting the statements in each chapter.   As a physician, I have nothing to gain by recommending everyone read *How Not To Die*, other than the sheer joy of knowing people will be able to become and stay well if they follow even half of the recommendations.

- Dr. Sal

A Comprehensive Approach to Balance Problems

Recently, I was visited in my office by a person with Parkinson's disease (PD) after he had fallen down the stairs. He told me that he falls a lot, so we spent some time talking about his battle with Parkinson's and the reason for his falls. Unfortunately, falling is a very common problem with Parkinson's disease, as well as many aging individuals with muscle weakness.

PD is a movement disorder. Because of changes that occur in a specific area of the brain, the individual may have difficulty starting to move. Once they get going, problems develop stopping the movements. Falls are common because of the difficulty stopping the movement and weakness in the lower extremities resulting in wobbly walking.

Scientists have defined the chemical imbalance related to PD. We know this is related to a problem with decreased production of dopamine in a specific area of the brain. The cause of this dopamine imbalance is unknown. One theory is that exposure to pesticides and other chemicals in the environment are at least associated with an increased risk, incidence of PD and other neurodegenerative disorders.

In the initial stage of PD, the symptoms are mild tremors or shaking of the hands. Posture can become rounded. Some individuals develop early problems with balance. Their friends and family might notice abnormal facial expressions. As symptoms progress, the individual develops problems with activities of daily living. Normal physical tasks become more problematic and the person might develop even more difficulty walking, even start to fall. In the latter stage, movements become slow and the individual has problems initiating movements. The limbs become more rigid and hard to move. In

260

addition to the musculoskeletal symptoms, the person might also develop problems with cognition. The brain function slows, adding to the problems with activities of daily living.

Other neurodegenerative disorders which affect activities of daily living include Alzheimer's dementia (AD), multiple sclerosis (MS) and strokes. AD is characterized by a progressive loss of mental function and has less musculoskeletal dysfunction. MS and strokes can affect limb function and may increase the risk of falling. MS is a troublesome disorder since the symptoms are intermittent and occur in different parts of the body at different times. The lesions of MS which occur in different parts of the brain and spinal cord produce variable symptoms such as numbness in an extremity at one time, speech problems another time or even vision problems yet another time. Symptoms are intermittent and the hallmark of the illness.

Strokes occur as a result of a blockage of blood flow to a specific part of the brain. In some cases, plaque develops in the carotid arteries (the large arteries which can be felt in the neck). If a piece of the plaque breaks loose, it travels into the arteries in the brain and lodges in a small vessel. The area of the brain supplied by this artery starts to die immediately, since it is not receiving proper blood, oxygen and nutrients. This is the reason the term stroke attack is used. Similar to a heart attack, the person affected by stroke symptoms should immediately call 911 and go by ambulance to the emergency room. While in the ambulance, the EMT professionals can administer medications which will help minimize brain cell death. They communicate with the ER physician and immediately start administering helpful therapies. As with PD, the chronic complications from a stroke can result in extremity weakness with an increased risk of falling.

The above information details several neurodegenerative illnesses which may increase the risk of falling and in time affect the individual's ability to perform activities of daily living. What can be done to help? Early risk factor identification is very important. This is another reason everyone should have an annual visit with their physician. Even when a person is feeling well, they might be having subtle signs or symptoms which clue the physician/health care provider of a specific problem. The symptoms might sound benign to the patient, yet might be a helpful sign to the physician that something is wrong. In this situation, early intervention is very important. Even if a specific diagnosis is not initially made, physical therapy can be started to help the person regain strength and decrease the risk of falling.

It is concerning to me when I hear patients talk about hip fractures in a cavalier way. Sometimes I hear them make statements that it is an easy fix when someone breaks their hip. You simply go to an orthopedic surgeon, have a hip replacement or surgery to repair the fracture and everything is back to normal. The statistics do not support this statement. Many people suffering from a hip fracture end up in a nursing home for an extended period of time after the surgery and many never regain their pre-fracture level of function. This indicates that complications of a hip fracture can be severe and is a reason a person with a balance problem needs immediate attention. There are certain physical therapists that specialize in balance disorders and referral to such an individual is helpful when the health care provider diagnoses a balance problem. The physical therapist might also work with an exercise specialist to help the individual regain lost muscle strength and/or function. A comprehensive approach to fall prevention helps the most. As detailed above, this includes the physician/nurse practitioner, a physical therapist trained in balance disorders, an exercise specialist and certainly the family and other care givers.

Recovery from a stroke or effective treatment of PD, AD or other neurodegenerative disorders requires a team approach that might include a psychologist, since many times the affected individual becomes very stressed, even depressed over the above mentioned illnesses. With a comprehensive team approach, the individual can look forward to the best possible outcome. For my patients with any of the above neurodegenerative disorders, I also include a nutrition evaluation and plan of action if the person is found to have a less than optimal nutritional status. It is very difficult to recover from any illness when the nutritional status is not optimal. Maximizing the nutritional content of the food a person eats adds to success in the comprehensive treatment approach.

- Dr. Sal

Kidneys ... What They Do For Us

The kidneys are two vital organs located underneath the rib cage just above the hip bone and towards the back. Picture someone putting their hands in the back pockets of their pants and you get an idea of where the kidneys are located. The kidneys function to filter the blood and excrete waste products via the urine (the kidneys feed urine into the bladder via small tubes called ureters). Kidneys regulate the amount of water in the body and control the levels of electrolytes. They function to maintain the critically important level of acid in the blood referred to as pH. Common waste products excreted by the kidneys include ammonium and urea yet, there are also dozens of chemicals, hormones and toxins filtered from the blood and excreted by the kidneys. The kidneys also help regulate the levels of glucose and amino acids (the building blocks for proteins). They produce hormones including calcitonin which helps regulate calcium balance and bone strength and erythropoietin that helps maintain normal red blood cell production. The kidneys produce and secrete renin, an enzyme for regulating normal blood pressure. The kidneys play a vital role in maintaining health and life. We can live with one kidney, not without two.

The kidneys work in conjunction with other organs in the body. One good example is the interplay of the kidneys with the lungs in maintaining acid-base balance. The lungs regulate carbon dioxide (CO_2) concentrations and the kidneys function to regulate the reabsorption of hydrogen ions (acid) and bicarbonate (base) chemicals in order to strictly control the acid-base balance. The kidneys also work in conjunction with the brain in specific areas called the hypothalamus and pituitary to regulate the amount of water in the body via a hormone called ADH. This hormone is released from the brain and travels in the blood to the kidneys altering the amount of water reabsorbed from specific areas of the kidneys. These are just a few examples of the intricate functions of the kidneys and how they interact with other parts of the body to keep us healthy.

Diseases which affect the kidneys include: nephritic and nephrotic syndromes, kidney cysts, acute kidney injury, urinary tract infections, kidney stones/obstruction and cancers. Some of these diseases result in chronic kidney damage and loss of function others are more acute and temporary. The kidneys, like other vital organs, have the ability to heal themselves if the damage is not too severe. One of the most common illnesses affecting the kidneys is diabetes, the leading cause of chronic kidney failure in the U.S. The term for this is diabetic nephropathy and results from years of damage to the kidneys from high blood glucose/hyperglycemia. During the initial years of diabetic kidney damage, there are few symptoms. As the disease progresses, kidney damage results in chronic fatigue, changes in urine volume, headaches, leg swelling and other signs of disease. Kidney damage alters water reabsorption and blood pressure resulting in hypertension (high blood pressure). In addition to the damage caused to the kidneys from the high levels of glucose in the blood, diabetes is one of the leading causes of blindness and amputations resulting from impaired circulation to the eyes and extremities. The arteries in the body become damaged by the high glucose which creates what are called Advanced Glycation End products (AGEs). Over the years, these AGEs damage the inner lining of the blood vessels and decrease blood flow to all areas of the body. This also occurs in the blood vessels of the heart resulting in Coronary Artery Disease (CAD). As a result, many diabetics suffer from heart attacks and strokes.

Kidney function is also affected by medications as well as any chemicals in the blood stream. Many medications are metabolized and excreted from the kidneys. They have the potential to cause damage to the kidneys when the levels of these medications are not well controlled. Doctors have the ability to monitor the levels of medications and their effect on the renal (kidney) function via simple blood tests. Common medications which can negatively affect renal function include antibiotics, statin medications for high cholesterol and many others, therefore, it is most helpful to err on the side of caution when taking any medication. The rule of thumb is to take a medication only when the benefits far outweigh the risks, take the lowest dose necessary to correct the problem being treated and monitor the effects of the medication on the kidneys, liver and body as a whole.

Besides the hundreds of medications which may affect the kidneys, there are thousands of environmental chemicals which also alter kidney function. On a daily basis we are bombarded by hundreds of chemicals in the water we drink, foods we eat, air we breathe and the grass we play on with our children. We clean our homes with chemicals and lather our bodies with tanning lotions, deodorants and perfumes – all chemicals that enter the body and then have to be metabolized and excreted by the kidneys and/or the liver. The reader begins to get a sense of how vital the kidneys are and how they work continuously to maintain good health.

How can we keep our kidneys healthy . . . one way is by drinking lots of clean water daily. There are various recommendations for how much to drink; commonly, people are told to drink 6-8 glasses per day which amounts to about 64 oz. One good way to know if you are drinking enough is to look at the color of the urine. If it is clear as opposed to dark yellow, you are probably drinking enough water. The skin also gives us other clues to the level of hydration. When you pinch the skin and then release it, the skin should quickly go back into its normal position if you are well hydrated. If you are deficient in water, the skin tents up and slowly returns to normal. Blood pressure will also be lower, and a person might complain of dizziness when not well hydrated. Low blood pressure from dehydration is not good for the kidneys or for health in general. This may cause a person to faint resulting in a host of other acute injuries.

It is important to have a wellness consultation annually. Your physician/health care provider can order blood and/or urine tests to measure the renal/kidney function. There is also ultrasound, x-ray, CT scans and MRI tests which can be done to further evaluate the anatomy and physiologic function of the kidneys. With the right tests, your physician can provide you with information vital to the health of your kidneys.

- Dr. Sal

What Are Tremors?

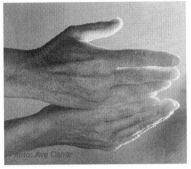

The definition of a tremor is an unintentional, rhythmic movement, a to-and-fro oscillation which usually occurs in the hands and fingers but may also involve the lower extremities, face or voice.

Tremors can occur at rest or with purposeful movement known as action tremors. Tremors can occur with Parkinson's disease, multiple sclerosis (MS), traumatic brain injury (TBI), strokes, chronic liver disease, brain tumors, metabolic disorders, alcoholism; and, toxins such as mercury, lead or arsenic. Tremors may also occur as a side effect of prescription medications and illicit drugs such as cocaine.

Tremors occur in about 25% of those with Parkinson's disease. PD is a movement disorder also characterized by loss of facial expression, slowness of speech and movement, gait abnormalities, stooped posture, stiffness of muscles, muscle pain and lack of dexterity. The tremors of PD often occur as a pill-rolling motion involving the thumb and first fingers, they can also occur as an eyelid flutter, a flickering of the jaw or lips. The PD tremor is described as a rest tremor which occurs when the person is at rest and the body is supported against gravity. Intentional movements often decrease the tremors associated with PD.

Tremors can also be associated with other neurologic diseases such as multiple sclerosis (MS), dementia and traumatic brain injury (TBI). MS is a neurologic condition that has variable signs and symptoms since the brain lesions appear in different areas of the central nervous system. Dementia has several forms including

268

Alzheimer's disease, vascular and Lewy body dementia. TBI occurs as a result of accidental injury to the brain; it is common in sports where repetitive head trauma occurs such as football, soccer, boxing and mixed-martial arts. In these situations, tremors can occur and vary in severity, frequency and description.

Tremors may occur with a variety of metabolic disorders including electrolyte abnormalities such as low sodium, calcium, glucose, magnesium; also, hyperthyroidism (high thyroid hormone levels), hyperparathyroidism (high parathyroid hormone levels) and advanced liver or kidney disease.

Psychogenic tremors (also called functional tremors) are usually sudden in onset, resolve quickly and appear to be associated with stress or emotional situations. They may be associated with specific psychological disorders. They often resolve quickly when the person is distracted.

Physiologic tremors occur in every normal individual and are rarely visible to the eye. They occur as a result of strong emotions, physical exhaustion, hypoglycemia (low blood sugar), hyperthyroidism, heavy metal poisoning (lead or mercury), stimulants (caffeine, cocaine), alcohol withdrawal, infections or fever. Physiologic tremors are often described as jitters and are generally not caused by a neurological disease but by a reaction to certain drugs, alcohol withdrawal, or medical conditions and are usually reversible once the cause is corrected.

Tremors may result from other conditions such as excessive alcohol consumption or withdrawal. Alcohol can kill certain nerve cells, resulting in tremors, especially in the hands. Interestingly, a small amount of alcohol may help decrease essential/benign tremors.

Tremors occur with diseases which injure the peripheral nerves – the nerves outside of the central nervous system. Peripheral neuropathy may occur when the nerves that supply the body's muscles are traumatized by injury or by diseases such as diabetes, B12 deficiency and thyroid abnormalities.

Various forms of dementia including vascular and multi-infarct may cause tremors. In this situation, multiple small infarcts occur in various areas of the brain that in time culminate in diffused brain dysfunction. An infarct occurs when blood supply to an area of the body is significantly decreased and the cells start to die (infarct). When this occurs in the brain, tremors and other symptoms can occur including all those we know as dementia. Multi-infarct dementia (MID) is a form of vascular disease and is associated with high blood pressure, high cholesterol, heart disease and diabetes. In all these conditions, the blood supply to the brain is diminished; tremors may occur in addition to other symptoms, including loss of memory and changes in personality.

Lewy body dementia is a degenerative neurologic condition where abnormal proteins called Lewy bodies accumulate in the brain destroying brain cells, predisposing the person to tremors, cognitive problems and progressive dementia.

Drug-induced tremors may occur with caffeine, cocaine, prescription stimulant medications, steroids, some anti-depressant and thyroid medications. Toxins which can cause brain damage and result in tremors include arsenic (which is found in many common foods and drinks), mercury (found in fish) and lead from lead-based paints (used in the past).

There are many reasons for tremors to occur. A person should seek medical attention when tremors are new and persistent over a few months, when they interfere with activities of daily living or become chronic. It is important to visit your primary care physician or a neurologist (a physician who specializes in diseases of the brain) for a diagnosis and treatment.

After the physician discusses the details of the tremors with the patient, a full examination will be done, including an extensive neurologic examination. Tests may be ordered including blood tests for glucose, electrolytes, B12, thyroid hormone, liver and kidney function. More specific tests may check the levels of toxins in the blood (arsenic, lead, mercury) and imaging tests might include CAT scans of the brain or an MRI. A spinal tap (lumbar puncture) may be required to take fluid from around the spinal cord. This test allows the pathologist to analyze the cells bathing the spinal cord and brain that may give evidence of multiple sclerosis (MS), Lewy body dementia or other chronic neurologic diseases.

Treatment of the tremors depends on the cause. Certainly, the patient will be counseled on limiting or avoiding alcohol and recreational drugs, talking with their physician to identify if the tremors are the result of any prescription medications the person is taking. If stress is a factor, a plan is made to deal with the stress. As with any other area of health, prevention is the best medicine and a plan should be made to keep the brain healthy. Learning something new each day, such as word games or puzzles, dancing or a new language may be suggested. Socialization is great for the brain as is healthy nutrition. In addition, regular physical activity has been proven to increase brain function.

- Dr. Sal

Exercise Versus Fitness Training

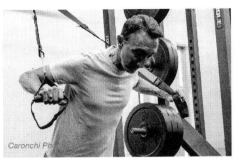

Caronchi Ph

While most people know the American Heart Association recommends 30 minutes of moderately intense physical exercise most days of the week, do most people know if this is doing any good? Many people are told by their doctor during their annual physical to exercise yet, how many people are formally tested for their baseline level of fitness before starting an exercise program? Also, how many people work with an exercise specialist to measure their progress? At a recent medical conference I attended, the speaker advised not starting treatment for high blood pressure without knowing the individual's baseline blood pressure and to regularly measure the response to treatment (a blood pressure medication in most cases) . . . so why don't we do this when we prescribe exercise? In most cases, we do not measure baseline fitness and the response to exercise to decide if the current exercise regimen is effective. If people are exercising while not progressing and getting fit and healthier, what is the purpose?

Exercise has many purposes and multiple benefits. Research shows that regular physical activity lowers blood pressure, improves cholesterol levels, decreases the risk of heart disease, improves insulin sensitivity, lowers the risk of diabetes, improves brain function and minimizes the risk of dementia. Exercise lessens the risk of most chronic illnesses, decreases mortality and improves longevity. With all these wonderful benefits (and almost no negative side effects) why are

272

we not more prescriptive about the exercise regimen? Why are we not doing more to measure baseline levels and the progression over time?

When it comes to measuring, how is this actually done? The answer is: Vo2 max. This is the maximum amount of oxygen the body is able to use to make energy. It is essentially a measure of cardio-respiratory fitness or, how well the heart and lungs do their job. The Vo2 max is measured when a person walks or runs on a treadmill. The individual's heart rhythm, blood pressure and oxygen levels are monitored during a 6-8 minute walk on a treadmill. The walking starts out slow and then progresses over the 6-8 minute period, as does the elevation of the treadmill. The test is stopped when the individual gets to about 80% of their calculated maximum, as determined by age. This is a very important number since an increase in Vo2 correlates with a decrease in the risk of death, cancer, diabetes and dementia. Regular physical activity has been shown to decrease the risk of Alzheimer's by 50% (Reference: *Alzheimer's Research & Prevention Foundation*).

Regular physical activity improves heart function by enabling the heart to pump more blood with each contraction. It enables the body to extract more oxygen from the red blood cells. It also increases the capillaries around the muscles which mean there are more blood vessels in the muscles bringing more oxygen and nutrients to the muscle cells. Finally, it increases the efficiency of the mitochondria, the parts of the cells where energy is made. To make the heart and circulatory system healthier, endurance exercise is better than strength training. The latter in many cases is associated with more periods of high blood pressure which strains the heart and can potentially result in ventricular hypertrophy. The main pumping chamber of the heart (the ventricle) becomes abnormally thickened, which is not healthy for the heart. If the goal is to improve heart function and lower blood pressure, endurance exercise wins out. How long do you need to exercise to get these benefits? Research shows that the higher the intensity of the exercise the more the benefit. High intensity exercise

273

is the best way to improve cardio-respiratory fitness. (References: *Journal of Applied Physiology* Dec 2014 and *JAMA* 2013 volume 309 section 2, page 143).

When starting an exercise plan, it is more important to initially focus on frequency – the number of times of exercise weekly. Once this is consistent, the exercise regimen focuses on the time the person is exercising, when the person is consistent with the amount of exercise, the prescription moves on to intensity. Studies have shown higher intensity produces more overall benefits and less time a person has to spend exercising.

The exercise prescription should include a deliberate schedule, a specific time allotted for each exercise session and measurements of progress documented. There should be a focus on weaknesses to concentrate on and attention paid to mindless repetition. The overall goal of exercise is to become healthier, fit and functional with emphasis on functional. If a person is able to walk 30 minutes on a treadmill yet has difficulty carrying a heavy bag of groceries up a flight of stairs, the exercise regimen must be reworked. Fitness and functionality lead to improved quality of life and longevity.

Even the sedentary person can benefit from regular physical activity by developing a schedule that allows consistent frequency of exercise. Increasing the time of each exercise session and the intensity will produce maximum benefits. Have a baseline measurement of Vo2 max and repeat every 6-12 months. Physical changes will become evident; your body will look more muscular and less flabby. Energy and sleep quality should improve. The level of overall fitness and well-being should be obvious. Aging will slow down — a sense of feeling younger and more vital. The action plan for the reader is to work with their physician and exercise specialist to develop a program as described above — enjoy all the benefits regular physical activity has to offer!

- Dr. Sal

Using Flaxseed as a Functional Food

Functional foods are those that provide specific health benefits over and above their nutritional value — flaxseed is a perfect example. Research has shown the health benefits of flaxseed in potentially lowering the risk of heart disease, obesity, diabetes and even some cancers. What is it about flaxseed that makes it such a healthful product? History shows that flaxseed is one of the oldest crops cultivated since the beginning of civilization. The technical term for flaxseed is *Linum usitatissimum*, meaning "very useful" in Latin. Every part of the flaxseed plant is used commercially. The stem yields high quality fibers used in clothing and has also been used to make paper. The flaxseed oil and some of its sub-products are used in animal feed.

As a functional food, flaxseed is important since it contains alpha linoleic acid (ALA), lignans and antioxidants. Alpha linoleic acid (ALA) is the precursor of DHA and EPA, also known as Omega-3 fatty acids (w3FAs) essential for the formation of cell membranes and the production of steroid hormones. In the cell membrane, these fatty acids keep the cells fluid and flexible. When ALA is converted to EPA and DHA, these chemicals are used by the cells resulting in less inflammation and thought to lower the risk of cardiovascular disease. Flaxseed is rich in poly-unsaturated fatty acids (PUFAs) that also help lower the risk of heart disease and strokes.

Lignans are found in most plants and are chemicals that act as antioxidants and called phytoestrogens. Inflammation is one of the causes of cardiovascular disease and many other chronic illnesses. Inflammation in the cells causes oxidation similar to rusting of the cells from within; antioxidants in plants help limit this process and

275

keep the cells healthier. Phytoestrogens are chemicals within plant cells that are structurally related to estrogen. These chemicals weakly bind to estrogen receptors and are thought to limit the negative health effects of estrogen. Studies by Tham, et al, have shown promising effects of flaxseed lignans, reducing the growth of cancerous tumors of the breast, prostate and endometrium.

Flaxseed also contains a healthy amount of protein and fiber. The protein content of flaxseed varies from 20-30%. Flaxseed amino acids, the building blocks for proteins, are similar to soybeans. They contain no gluten protein (the type of protein causing celiac disease). Many people use flaxseed in their foods, baked goods, salads and smoothies to increase the overall amount of protein in the diet.

Flaxseed fibers are among the oldest crops in the world; the use of flax in the production of linen dates back to ancient Egyptian times. Flax fiber is also used in the production of high quality paper, printed banknotes and the rolling paper for cigarettes and teabags.

Flaxseed contains healthy amounts of potassium, calcium, magnesium and phosphorous. These minerals are helpful to maintaining health of bones and keeping blood pressure normal. As a medicinal product, flaxseed has been used for Ayurvedic healing in India, Sri Lanka, China and other countries for centuries. It is thought to bring mental and physical endurance by fighting fatigue and slowing the aging process. Wound healing has also been thought to be the result of flaxseed, increasing the production of prostaglandins via the omega-3 fatty acids mentioned above. The flaxseed provides the omega-3 fatty acids; the body uses it to produce these prostaglandin substances for wound healing. During the middle ages, flaxseed was used to treat various gastrointestinal disorders, as a diuretic in the treatment of kidney problems, for pain relief and the treatment of some tumors. The medicinal benefits of flaxseed are described in the writings of Hippocrates and in various textbooks on medicinal herbs used in Europe and Asia over the centuries.

In the treatment of diabetes, flaxseed may be helpful since the flaxseed lignans decrease the function of a gene that produces an enzyme responsible for the synthesis of glucose (sugar) in the liver. The PRASAD project (Philanthropic Relief, Altruistic Service & Development) in 2002 supplemented diabetic patients with flaxseed for one month; it resulted in a 19.7% reduction in blood glucose and a 15.6% reduction in the A1C blood tests (a measure of the blood sugar control) over a three month period. Research done by Woodside in 2006 and Chen in 2011 showed that adding flaxseed to the diet might lower the level of insulin and IGF-1. Lower amounts of insulin in the body are obviously helpful in diabetes; and, a lower level of IGF-1 is believed to help decrease the risk of various cancers. The other anti-cancer mechanism flaxseed is thought to provide is by the production of enterodiol and enterolactone (plant estrogens) that block some of the effects of estrogen and limit its negative, cancer-causing effects. This research was done by Penttinen in 2007.

Research done by Cicero and others, in 2010, showed the omega-3 fatty acids provided by flaxseed lowered blood pressure and helped in the treatment of individuals with chronic kidney disease. The other chronic disease that flaxseed helps with is cardiovascular disease. Since flaxseed is high in fiber, it actually decreases the GI absorption of cholesterol from the diet. Mohamed, in 2012, showed improvement in lipid profiles of patients with diabetes supplemented with flaxseed for two months. In the treatment of obesity, flaxseed is helpful since it slows gastric emptying and decreases the absorption of calories. Since flaxseed binds a lot of water in the GI tract producing a thick fluid, it also produces satiety and suppresses the appetite.

Flaxseed is a healthful, functional food providing the omega-3 fatty acid ALA as well as antioxidants that help in decreasing the risk of cardiovascular disease, fiber to improve GI function and lignans that have been shown to potentially decrease cancer cell growth. One third cup of raw flaxseed can be added to salads, smoothies, cereal or baked goods daily for the intended benefits.   - Dr. Sal

277

Can Telomeres Determine Your Age?

In researching clinical literature for an anti-aging presentation, I read Elizabeth Blackburn's book, *The Telomere Effect*, which I highly recommend. This book gives insight into how we age and what we can do to slow the process. Telomeres are the protective ends of the chromosomes – the parts of all cells that contain our DNA and genes. Dr. Blackburn explains the telomeres are similar to the protective plastic tips on shoelaces. These plastic tips keep the shoelaces from unraveling; the telomeres within our cells have a similar function to protect the chromosomes from changing shape and becoming less functional. The telomeres protect the chromosomes, the DNA and the genes that enable us to remain healthy.

With age, the telomeres shorten making the chromosomes more susceptible to damage. When the telomeres get to a certain length, the cells start to die; this is one of the theories on how we age. With short telomeres, the chromosomes are more susceptible to damage from UV radiation from the sun, environmental toxins in food, water and air, possibly from infections and other unknown insults. The length of the telomeres can be measured yet, does this give an accurate measurement of a person's physiologic age? The answer is yes, partially. The length of the telomeres gives some information about the internal age of a person, however, there are many other things that can be measured.

All cells in the body make energy in the form of ATP and cannot survive without it. Energy (ATP) is made in the parts of the cells called the mitochondria, considered the powerhouse of the cells. Mitochondrial dysfunction or decline is another theory of aging. It is believed that the things mentioned above that may potentially damage

278

the telomeres may also damage the mitochondria, therefore, the cell's ability to make energy. Similar to automobiles when they run out of gas, the engine stops running. When the cells are unable to make ATP, they no longer function; the cells begin to die and the organ these cells make up begins to die.

Another theory of aging relates to the dozens of hormones we produce. As we age, hormone production decreases. In females, estrogen and progesterone decline; in males, testosterone declines. In addition, all other hormones made by the various endocrine cells in the body decline, with the exception of the stress hormone, cortisol. Without normal hormone levels, the body is unable to perform the normal physiologic functions resulting in problems with sleep, cognition, heart function, blood pressure, temperature regulation and other problems. As a whole, the body ages more rapidly when hormone levels decline and are not supplemented. In my practice, when symptoms dictate, I have the individual do either blood or saliva tests to measure the various hormones and we make an action plan based on the results. Often I refer the individual to an integrative/ functional medicine specialist for further hormone therapy.

Next, there is the toxin mediated theory of aging. Over the past 100 years there has been the introduction of 85,000 chemicals into the world. On a daily basis we are bombarded by hundreds of chemicals: in foods, water, liquids, air, lotions, insecticides, herbicides and pesticides. These environmental toxins are unavoidable; the greater the exposure, the greater the potential damage to our cells and health. Many of these chemicals are called endocrine disruptors since they negatively affect the hormone balance in the cells making the individual susceptible to cancer, many chronic illnesses and more rapid aging.

Another theory of aging has to do with nutrition. If we use the automobile analogy, putting cheap gas in a car engine makes the engine run less efficiently; putting cheap (unhealthy) food/drinks into your body makes your cells function less efficiently. Nutrient deficiencies are also thought to accelerate the aging process because the cells do not have the vitamins, minerals, antioxidants and other chemicals needed to carry on with the thousands of chemical reactions that occur every day. The standard American diet consists of proteins laced with unnatural hormones, antibiotics, pesticides and fecal material. The carbohydrates many people eat are processed and high in sugar. The fats are often trans fats, chemically modified fats, directly contributing to heart disease, strokes and dementia.

While there are many reasons why we age, we all do not age at the same rate. We may see other individuals our own age, some who look younger and some older. The reason this happens is often related to the lifestyle of the individual. Genetics does play a role yet, we know from many clinical studies that healthy lifestyle behaviors can keep bad genes turned off — a healthy lifestyle can turn on good healthy genes!

As mentioned above, we are able to measure telomere length to get an indication of the person's internal age; it may be more accurate if a person is aging rapidly to look at their skin, listen to how they live, making an overall assessment of their lifestyle and health risks. This is one reason I recommend my patients have an annual wellness/lifestyle visit. This enables the physician to understand the individual's risk factors for chronic disease and cancer who can then work with them to develop a healthy living action plan. A typical healthy living action plan would include: limiting or avoiding environmental toxins, developing a healthy eating action plan, scheduling time for exercise daily, limiting stress, getting enough quality sleep, having a purpose in life – a reason to get out of bed in the morning.

- Dr. Sal

Lifestyle Medicine . . . Changing the Health of the Nation

After many years of delivering traditional internal medical care, in 2010 I fortunately transitioned into a branch of health care that is changing the health of the nation. Traditional health care focuses on the care of sick people. This is the reason many people believe we have a sick care system, not a health care system. Traditional health care providers deal with the symptoms, attempting to cure rather than prevent disease. This type of health care focuses on the end of the pathologic process (disease reversal) rather than on the early development of disease, working with the individual to institute significant lifestyle behavior change. The majority of chronic illnesses and cancers people suffer from are the result of unhealthy living. A change in lifestyle results in less risk, less incidence of chronic disease and cancer. Many research studies have proven these points.

My transition and thought process, as well as the paradigm shift in my clinical practice, came before I accepted a new role at Lee Health. Over 20 years of practicing internal medicine, I have encouraged patients to adopt a healthy lifestyle. Since 2010, my focus has been on doing this as the System Medical Director of Wellness & Employee Health. The former name, Lee Memorial Health System, was changed to Lee Health to communicate that we are *Caring People, Inspiring Health*. This mission statement is meant to help people understand our goal to help individuals become and stay healthy. We want to keep people healthy, rather than getting sick requiring hospital care. Hippocrates stated as the first tenet of medicine, *Do no harm*. As medical professionals, we must do all we can to help people avoid illness, following the Hippocrates' principle. This is why I love practicing preventive medicine; it focuses on wellness rather that sickness.

Over the years, I have realized that lifestyle modification is a perfect part of the treatment and reversal plan. Many of my patients have developed a chronic illness, then reverse their disease after intensive lifestyle behavior modification. I have witnessed this often in patients with cardiovascular disease, high blood pressure, diabetes and many inflammatory illnesses. Clinical research and many anecdotal reports reveal the power of healthy nutrition and healthy living. In the past seven years, my clinic has morphed into a lifestyle management practice. Since 2010, I have visited over 700 patients, sometimes desperate, looking for advice on how to become and stay well. Many have had significant weight problems. Others have had many risk factors for chronic disease and cancer. Invariably for almost all, I ask them to tell me the specifics of their diet in an attempt to understand if they eat the CRAP-SAD diet (calorie-rich and processed standard American diet) or, if they eat more plant-based, nutritious foods. During the initial visit, I usually find that most of the folks who come to see me eat the former; that is when I tell them about the power of plants. I emphasize the tremendous health benefits of a whole food, plant-based diet and discuss how processed foods promote disease.

We also talk about the health benefits of being physically active, minimizing stress, getting enough quality sleep, knowing what they are passionate about, having a purpose in life. During the time we spend together at the initial visit and later sessions, we talk extensively about the major influence lifestyle has over genetics explaining that even when a person inherits bad genes, the individual has the power to keep these bad genes turned off by living a healthy life. I emphasize health has to be the number one priority each day when getting out of bed. I mention that failing health causes all other priorities to also fail; instead, a person can achieve so much in life when they remain healthy.

My role as System Medical Director of Wellness and Employee Health is to work on motivating people to see the benefits explained above. In this role I have the responsibility to be a coach, advocate, role model, teacher, health care quarterback and a teammate. I emphasize that the patient and the physician should function as a team (with other health care providers, family members and friends) to develop a healthy living action plan. This plan should be developed to move closer to the most important health care goals.

I have been working for Lee Health for over 26 years and am proud to be a part of the team of dedicated health care providers and administrators. I have seen significant changes in how the leaders of this health system think and act to provide the best health care possible. In recent years, I have seen how the lifestyle medicine approach to health care has gained support and how products and services have been developed to improve the health of over 19,000 employees and dependents on our health plan. As a self-insured company, Lee Health has a vested interest in keeping these folks healthy, knowing that its employees are its most valuable asset. Healthier employees are more productive, efficient and effective health care providers. Employees are more compassionate if they are not dealing with their own health care problems allowing them to focus on the health of the patients.

When I first started to practice internal medicine in 1993, the focus was (and still is, in many cases) on treating the symptoms and trying to cure disease. There has been a paradigm shift in recent years — not just in thinking, but also in actions. Many health care providers now focus on the cause of the disease to help individuals avoid disease through risk factor modification. Many physicians and health care systems have now incorporated what in the past was termed complementary and alternative medicine (CAM). We know that traditional medical care consists of prescription medications, procedures and surgery. Not all people need these to resolve a health care problem. Many times, a change in lifestyle is all that is needed.

Even when traditional medical approaches are necessary, the addition of lifestyle medicine makes traditional health care more effective. Examples of this are seen daily when treating people for diabetes, high blood pressure, high cholesterol, osteoarthritis, to name a few.

Since 2012, I have been involved in the CHIP program (Complete Health Improvement Program). This is a nine-week program run by a facilitator who teaches people about the tremendous power of plant-based nutrition. In a classroom session the facilitator works with groups of about 25-30 individuals teaching how to shop, store, cook and enjoy plant-based foods. The facilitator helps the participants understand the importance of nutrition in health. I chaired a committee, Food is Medicine, and in these meetings, I taught similar concepts to physicians and other health care providers encouraging them to use lifestyle modification for all patients. The name of this committee has been changed to Lifestyle is Medicine, as we are now focusing on the importance of lifestyle in relation to health promotion and disease avoidance.

As I work with physicians, nurse practitioners and other health care providers, I continue to be struck by the overall lack of education in the area of lifestyle medicine. Even the medical residents graduating now are not learning what they need to know to incorporate lifestyle medicine into their daily work with patients. This is very unfortunate since many research articles have been published in national, peer reviewed journals showing the power of lifestyle medicine. Some physicians, myself included, have decided to learn on our own. I completed a certification program in Anti-Aging Medicine through A4M (American Academy of Anti-Aging Medicine) and a certification in lifestyle medicine through the American College of Lifestyle Medicine (ACLM). In addition, I have attended many conferences put on by A4M, ACLM, PCRM (Physicians Committee for Responsible Medicine) and the Plantrician Project. I have learned from the national leaders in this field including: Dr. Caldwell Esselstyn, Dr. Joel Fuhrman, Dr. Neal Barnard, Dr. Colin Campbell,

Dr. Hans Diehl, Dr. Scott Stoll, Dr. Marc Braman, Dr. Michael Greger, Dr. Philip Tuso, Brendan Brazier, and more – many have visited Lee Health to lecture to our medical staff and our community neighbors.

What I have learned over the past years by focusing on lifestyle medicine is not only is this a paradigm shift in how health care is delivered, it is a health care revolution. Traditional health care is strongly influenced by the pharmaceutical companies and agribusiness. The health of Americans over the past 50 years continues to decline as a result of unhealthy processed foods and lifestyles. We have become a pill-driven society and a fast-food nation. This has resulted in Americans spending more money on health care while getting far less than optimal health care outcomes. It is time to find a better way to deliver health care; I strongly believe the lifestyle medicine approach to health care is the answer. Over the coming years, I plan to devote my time and effort to advancing the specialty of lifestyle medicine. The focus needs to be on teaching medical professionals and the public about the power of this approach. Through awareness, education and action, we can change the world — I am humbled to play a small role in this transition.

- Dr. Sal

A Man is Only as Old as His Arteries

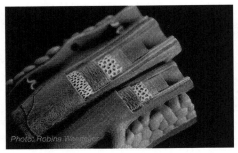
Photo: Robina W...

To quote the English physician, Thomas Sydenham (1624-1689), "A man is only as old as his arteries." He was certainly ahead of his time as we now know arterial aging is one of the mechanisms for chronic illnesses . . . heart attacks, strokes, dementia, erectile dysfunction and more.

Plaque formation develops early in adulthood as revealed by many autopsies performed on men who died in earlier wars. As plaque forms in the arterial wall, the flexibility of the arteries diminishes; the arteries become stiff, the pressure within the arteries increases and this places a strain on the heart that may lead to heart failure, if not treated. As plaque builds up, normal blood flow decreases; if a piece of the plaque comes lose, it flows down and eventually reaches the smallest blood vessel. This blocks blood flow to the organ it supplies, causing damage known as a heart attack when it involves the heart or a stroke involving the brain.

The causes of arterial aging include inflammation, oxidative stress and immune dysfunction. Inflammation occurs as a result of high cholesterol, toxins within the blood, elevated sugar, high blood pressure and more. Inflammation starts the process of plaque buildup; if not treated, the plaque increases resulting in the events described above.

Oxidation (think of how metal rusts when left in the rain) occurs when the body is exposed to stress of any kind whether from mental stress, elevated cortisol, heavy metal toxins in the blood or poor nutrition with a lack of antioxidants.

Immune dysfunction happens as a result of the body being exposed to toxins in the food, water, air and the environment. It may also be a result of chronic infections, hormone imbalance or deficiencies of essential vitamins, minerals and other nutrients.

These three mechanisms (inflammation, oxidative stress and immune dysfunction) all affect the ability of the arteries to make nitric oxide essential to maintaining normal, healthy arteries. Nitric oxide is a vasodilator, meaning it dilates/enlarges the arteries so blood flows easily.

High blood pressure injures the inner lining of the arteries (the endothelium). When this occurs and the endothelial cells lining the inner part of the arteries are damaged, the production of nitric oxide decreases; and, the arteries cannot dilate as they should.

Research has shown that the bacteria in the mouth help make and recycle nitric oxide and play a role in either maintaining normal blood pressure or in the development of hypertension (high blood pressure). *The Systolic Blood Pressure Intervention Trial* (SPRINT) showed that decreasing the systolic blood pressure (the top number in the blood pressure reading) from 140 down to 120 decreases the risk of heart attacks, heart failure and strokes by 1/3 and decreases the risk of death by 1/4.

In addition to lowering blood pressure, nitric oxide also functions to keep other areas of the body healthy by ensuring normal blood flow through the arteries to all cells in every organ. Without nitric oxide, the red blood cells would not be able to carry oxygen; if this did not happen, life would cease. It is important to realize that endothelial dysfunction is a process. In a newborn, the arteries are completely healthy yet soon after birth the child is exposed to all the things mentioned above that start making the arteries unhealthy. As this occurs throughout life, the production of nitric oxide decreases and the cells throughout the body begin to age.

Researchers have also shown that oral hygiene negatively affects the production of nitric oxide. Bacteria in the mouth chemically alter nitrates to nitrites which are eventually chemically changed into nitric oxide. Brushing the tongue and using lots of mouthwash can kill the very bacteria needed to make nitric oxide. In one study, one week of chlorhexidine mouthwash produced a 26 mmHg rise in blood pressure in those participating in this research!

Please don't misunderstand. We need to keep the mouth clean from pathogenic/disease producing bacteria. This is essential for the health of the teeth/gums and the health of the heart. Pathogenic bacteria in the mouth can get into the bloodstream and attach to cells in the heart causing damage. We need to keep the mouth clean, while at the same time, not so clean that we remove the essential bacteria. Stomach acid is involved in the process where nitrate is converted to nitrite and then to nitric oxide, therefore, getting rid of stomach acid makes it harder for the body to make nitric oxide. Since many people use medications to fight heartburn that decreases stomach acidity, the individual has a decreased ability to make nitric oxide.

One healthy source of dietary nitrates is vegetables. This is probably the reason we see a blood pressure lowering effect of diets that recommend lots of vegetables. For the reader interested in reading more about this, the reference is in the journal *Hypertension* 2015 Feb; 65(2):320-327 authored by Dr. Vikas Kapil. Specific foods high in dietary nitrates include spinach, broccoli, celery, cabbage and even lettuce. The amount depends on where the vegetables are grown. There is significant geographic variability, since the soil in different areas of the country contains different nutrients. Nonetheless, eating more veggies and some fruits daily increases dietary nitrates, allowing the body to make more nitric oxide.

Since high blood pressure injures the endothelial lining of the arteries and decreases nitric oxide levels, we must pay close attention to individuals with hypertension as this is the #1 risk factor for cardiovascular disease. In America, two-thirds of the population have either pre-hypertension (SBP 120-139) or have hypertension (SBP > 140); of those, 50% are on medications but not at their goal blood pressure. This means treatment is not effective to lower the pressure to a level that lowers the risk of heart attacks, heart failure, strokes and kidney problems. In a report from *Health Technology Assessment* 2003: 7(31): 1-94, a decrease of only 5 mmHg in the systolic blood pressure decreased the risk of strokes by 34% and the risk of heart disease by 21%.

In summary, we must decrease the age of the arteries by lowering the blood pressure. One way to do this is by eating 5-6 servings of high nitrate vegetables daily. Also, keep the mouth clean, yet not too clean. Exercise lowers blood pressure, reduces stress and improves sleep. All of the lifestyle behaviors written about not only lower blood pressure and the risk of disease, they also improve the quality and longevity of life. For more information on this subject, I refer the reader to the SPRINT trial as well as the website www.sciencedirect.com.

- Dr. Sal

More on the Science of Nutrition

Recently, I listened to a short podcast from Dr. Mark Hyman, Chairman for the Institute for Functional Medicine, "Dairy: Six reasons why you should avoid it at all costs," during which he basically says – listen to the message, I'm just the messenger. In my *News-Press* articles and during my public presentations, I have advocated the same to focus on the science of nutrition and not the messenger. Dr. Hyman speaks of the advertising slogan from the milk industry, "Got Milk?" and states, "Everyone knows you need to drink milk to be healthy, right?" He then answers, "Not necessarily." He explains the nutritional science involving dairy. He states that as a scientist, I have to look at what we know about dairy and then we use this information to make the best decisions to positively influence our health.

Dr. Hyman references the USDA Food Pyramid which currently recommends drinking three glasses of milk per day and goes on to talk about the scientific evidence that is counter to this recommendation. He explains that the USDA recommendation is not based on strict science. Some of the USDA committee members who recommend this actually work for the dairy industry — bringing up concern about a conflict of interest.

Dr. Hyman references Dr. Walter Willett, head of nutrition at the Harvard School of Public Health, one of the most vocal critics of the USDA food pyramid, calling it "udderly ridiculous!" When we study the science of nutrition, there are many concerns with recommending that humans drink cow's milk. First, cow's milk in its natural form is produced to fatten up baby calves. Anecdotal and clinical research reports show that children and adults who consume more dairy have more problems with being overweight and have a higher risk of osteoporosis, vascular disease, diabetes, allergies and asthma. The cow's milk which humans consume is not natural. It is highly processed and contaminated.

One myth to dispel is the need to drink milk and consume dairy to get calcium for strong bones. This is a myth because in addition to the calcium, milk also contains hormones, pesticides, bacteria, antibiotics and IGF-1, known to increase the risk of cancer. *The Nurses' Health Study* looked at the risk and incidence of osteoporosis and found women who consumed high amounts of dairy had more, not less, bone fractures. In reality, dairy weakens bones. Compare the rates of osteoporosis in the U.S. with Africa and Asia where people consume much less dairy and you find less osteoporosis.

Another problem with focusing just on calcium in relation to bone health is that the science actually shows calcium alone is not as bone protective as once thought. Vitamin D has actually been found to be more critical in building healthy bones. In my clinic at Lee Health, I measured the Vitamin D levels in patients coming in for their wellness examinations and found the far majority with either insufficient or fully deficient levels. I recommend an over-the-counter supplement of Vitamin D3. Also, I advise my patients get more calcium from dark green, leafy vegetables, providing a wide variety of health promoting vitamins, minerals, antioxidants and fiber.

In addition to the above, dairy has been linked to breast and prostate cancer risk probably due to a component in dairy called IGF-1 (Insulin Like Growth factor – 1). When elevated, this is known to stimulate the growth of cancer cells.

Other problems with dairy consumption include lactose intolerance and an exacerbation of irritable bowel syndrome (IBS). Many adults have lactose intolerance because as they age, they stop producing lactase, the enzyme needed to digest lactose, the milk protein. This causes an upset stomach and problems with gas, bloating and loose bowel movements. In addition, for individuals who already suffer from IBS, dairy often makes their symptoms worse.

In the U.S. and many developed countries, cardiovascular disease (CVD) is the number one cause of premature death and disability. Milk and dairy contain high amounts of saturated fat that directly contributes to CVD. In this situation, many people switch to low-fat cow's milk without realizing that although some of the fat has been removed, large amounts of sugar have been added thereby increasing the individual's risk for obesity and diabetes. So, what has been accomplished by this change? Nothing other than increasing the chance of one disease over another!

The Federal Trade Commission (FTC) previously asked the USDA to look into the scientific findings and health claims associated with the diary industry's milk mustache ads. The FTC was essentially asking the "Got Milk" industry, "Got proof?" What was found was contrary to the messages delivered by these ads. Milk does not improve sports performance. It increases the risk of the many illnesses and several cancers (breast and prostate in particular).

In addition to the research done by Drs. Hyman and Willett, another authority on the negative health effects of dairy is Dr. Neal Barnard, President of the Physicians Committee for Responsible Medicine. His book, *The Cheese Trap*, is highly recommended since it is loaded with scientific facts, all the supporting research to help the reader understand how unhealthy it is to consume dairy. As Dr. Hyman states in his video blog – sorry to be such a critic of dairy but as physicians, we are responsible to help patients understand the facts about nutrition. We are responsible for weeding out the myths and focus on what real scientific data proves. We must use the best knowledge available to make decisions about what to put in our bodies. Food consumption is probably the number one behavior influencing health and because most people eat three times a day, correct information must be available.

Nutritional science has proven that eating whole foods and avoiding processed foods leads to better health and increased longevity. The facts are clear and the science is valid. Dr. Michael Greger adds more to support these facts than probably any other physician. His website www.nutritionfacts.org is filled with literally thousands of clinical research articles detailing the health benefits of eating whole foods that we know helps treat, reverse and PREVENT disease. Got Proof? – Yes, I certainly do!

- Dr. Sal

Man-Made Illnesses

In the early 1900s most people died as a result of infectious illnesses. Fortunately, with improvements in sanitation, many of those illnesses have been eradicated. The illnesses that people die from today have a commonality; many are man-made illnesses, with heart disease being number one. The correct term used for heart disease should be vascular disease as for the most part the term heart disease is used to describe coronary artery disease (CAD) that represents blockage in the blood vessels supplying the heart. When a person has blockages in the arteries of the heart, they most likely have blockages in other arteries in the body. That is why a person diagnosed with CAD often has peripheral artery disease (PAD -- blockages in the arteries in the legs) and/or carotid artery stenosis (CAS -- blockages in the carotid arteries) that can be felt by pressing on the side of the neck which supplies the brain with blood. So, the term heart disease should be called vascular disease as this is a total body problem.

Endothelial dysfunction is the correct term used to explain why vascular disease occurs. Endothelial dysfunction (ED) occurs when the inner lining of the arteries become inflamed and unable to function normally. Inflammation is the root cause of many chronic, man-made illnesses such as dementia, CAD, PAD, CAS and even erectile dysfunction (the other ED). Systemic (total body) inflammation also occurs with most of the musculoskeletal diseases such as osteoarthritis, rheumatoid arthritis, fibromyalgia and degenerative joint disease.

Because inflammation appears to be the common denominator in most of the chronic illnesses many people in America suffer and die from each year, we need to ask the question: *why does this inflammation occur in the first place?* The simple answer in most cases is lifestyle. Over the last one-hundred years, we have created the American lifestyle we know has led to more disease, disability and death than anyone in the early part of the 20th century would have believed. Americans have progressed in many ways; except from a health perspective, we have regressed tremendously. Certainly, health care has advanced when we look at the success of prescription medications and surgical procedures. We have regressed on health care in the home. Personal responsibility for maintaining one's health seems to be at an all-time low. Many people would prefer to take a pill for high blood pressure or high cholesterol or have their gallbladder removed, rather than treat the cause of their hypertension, hyperlipidemia or gall bladder disease. Is it easier to swallow a pill rather than swallow some spinach — certainly, it is in the short term! There are long-term complications of not dealing with the root cause of the problem. Taking a pill or having one's gallbladder removed simply treats the symptoms. To cure a problem, you must eliminate the cause which in most cases is related to lifestyle. The standard American lifestyle consists of an unhealthy diet, very limited exercise, too much stress, not enough sleep and a lack of personal responsibility for one's health care.

The system we have in the U.S. and most developed nations today is a sick care system, not a health care system. On a daily basis medical professionals deal with: complications of high blood pressure (strokes and kidney failure), high cholesterol (heart attacks, strokes and dementia), diabetes (blindness, kidney failure and amputations), tobacco (lung and bladder cancer), eating too many red and processed meats (colon cancer) and obesity. These are primarily man-made diseases that were not a significant problem in the early 1900s. Since then they have become epidemic! The Center for Disease Control & Prevention (CDC) website shows a map of the U.S. for the past 25 years detailing the rise in obesity across the nation. Very few states in the U.S. 25 years ago had a significant problem with obesity — now ALL states in the union have an obesity rate over

33%! In this short period of time, over one-third of the population has become obese and the number of those in America who are overweight is over 60%! If you track the rise in all chronic illnesses, weight increased as did the incidence of diabetes, heart disease, cancer and musculoskeletal illnesses.

This coincides with a decline in healthy lifestyles in America. We have man-made our health problems. The good news is, we can resolve these problems with a commitment to a healthier lifestyle. Yes, we can treat, reverse and even prevent these illnesses from occurring in the first place! We must make health the #1 priority each day. As an Internal Medicine specialist, working with individuals and families on preventive health maintenance, I have seen numerous patients change their priorities once they become sick or are diagnosed with a chronic disease. It is sad to see the limited concern for health and health care many people have while living the standard American lifestyle only to develop an obsession for healthy living after being diagnosed with a chronic illness or cancer.

We get only one life. The key is to add not only years to life but life to the years we have. Most people in America spend the last ten years of their lives in sickness. The goal should be to spend the last years of life in wellness, growing older while maintaining vitality and functionality. The best way to die would be to die of old age similar to the way people die in the Blue Zone® areas of the world (Okinawa, Loma Linda, Sardinia, Costa Rica and Ikaria). In these areas there are more centenarians than any place else in the world with their commonality being a healthy lifestyle.

- Dr. Sal

About the Author

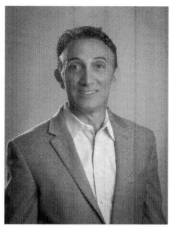

Caronchi Photography

Dr. Sal Lacagnina, D.O. is a graduate of NYCOM, The New York College of Osteopathic Medicine. He completed his Internal Medicine residency at the State University of New York at Stony Brook before coming to Florida in 1993 to join a private practice.

Shortly thereafter, Dr. Sal, as he likes to be called, was recruited by the Lee Memorial Health System where he practiced Internal Medicine and then became the Medical Director for the Lee Physician Group. Dr. Sal later became the Vice President for Health and Wellness and was later promoted to the System Medical Director for Employee Health at Lee Health.

In April 2020 Dr. Sal left Lee Health and started Concierge Lifestyle Medicine, a private practice in Fort Myers focusing on the Six Pillars of Lifestyle Medicine. This was a dream come true because Dr. Sal's passion focuses on the delivery of preventive health care.

Dr. Sal has been the author of a weekly health and wellness article in The News-Press since 2013. He lectures extensively throughout Florida and nationally on all topics related to health, wellness and preventive medicine.

Dr. Sal serves as the Medical Director for LMI, the Lifestyle Medicine Institute, which runs CHIP, the Complete Health Improvement Program and serves as an advisor for The Plantrician Project. Dr. Sal is also the President of HealthCentric.ai, an innovating company integrating computer generated technology into traditional health care in order to free up physicians and other providers to do the work they were trained to do. The automated intelligent electronic medical record system improves clinical outcomes, helps individuals with self-care and remote patient monitoring and is revolutionizing the delivery of medical care via ai - automated intelligence. HealthCentric.ai is a game-changer in delivering the highest quality healthcare.

Dr. Sal is board certified in Anti-Aging and Regenerative Medicine and is a Diplomate of the American College of Lifestyle Medicine.

Personally, Dr. Sal enjoys running, biking, tennis and all things outdoors. He also loves learning about his family heritage in Sicily, Italy.

Dr. Sal is the father of three children, the youngest of whom is 12 years of age and is helping to keep him young in body and spirit!

Affiliations:
Board Certified in Anti-Aging & Regenerative Medicine by The American Academy of Anti-Aging Medicine
Board Certified in Lifestyle Medicine by The American Board of Lifestyle Medicine
Board of Directors Member, American College of Lifestyle Medicine
Medical Director for Lifestyle Medicine Institute (CHIP Program)
The Plantrician Project, Advisory Board Member
President, HealthCentric.ai-US

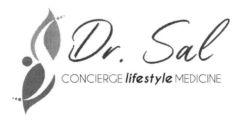

www.drsallifestylemed.com